EXTRAORDINARY ACHIEVEMENT

How To Get To The Next Level Of Success In Business *AND* Life

A Guide For Private Practice Entrepreneurs

By Paul Gough

Brought to you by

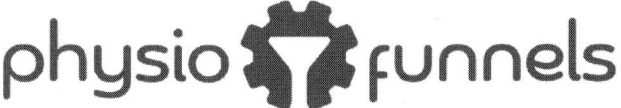

Copyright © 2023 Paul Gough. All rights reserved.

This publication is licensed to the individual reader only. Duplication or distribution by any means, including email, disk, photocopy, and recording, to a person other than the original purchaser, is a violation of international copyright law.

Publisher: Paul Gough, 25 Raby Road, Hartlepool, UK, TS24 8AS

While they have made every effort to verify the information here, neither the author nor the publisher assumes any responsibility for errors in, omissions from, or a different interpretation of the subject matter. This information may be subject to varying laws and practices in different areas, states, and countries. The reader assumes all responsibility for use of the information.

The author and publisher shall in no event be held liable to any party for any damages arising directly or indirectly from any use of this material. Every effort has been made to accurately represent this product and its potential and there is no guarantee that you will earn any money using these techniques.

ISBN: 9798861909648

Ready For Marketing To Get Easier?

If You Are A Private Practice Owner And You Are...

- Always wondering when this marketing thing will "get easier"...

- Fed up with doing the same old time-suck marketing that doesn't produce the type of new leads and clients you want?

- Sick of hearing your staff tell you they don't like to sell or say they don't have time to call new leads?

- Frustrated with not knowing if your marketing is working...

- **Fed up with having a bad website that costs money** (but doesn't produce anything in the way of new leads and perfect patients?)

- Confused about paying lots of money for a CRM that you only use 10% of *(that is STILL complicated years later?)*

- **Losing time** *(and money)* **having to use multiple different software to organize your marketing and sales follow up funnels?**

Announcing...

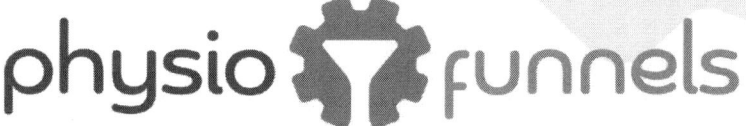

"The Marketing And Sales Automation Software That Helps Private Practice Owners SCALE With Ease"

Get A Completely FREE DEMO Of This New AI-Powered Technology At:

www.physiofunnels.com

For Your Consideration When You've Finished Reading The Book...

The 2-Day
EXTRAORDINARY ACHIEVEMENT
IN-PERSON WORKSHOP

"If you like what you read in this book, and you want to continue the journey, why not attend the **TOTAL IMMERSION** two-day event and work personally with Paul Gough to implement these life enhancing principles into your life?"

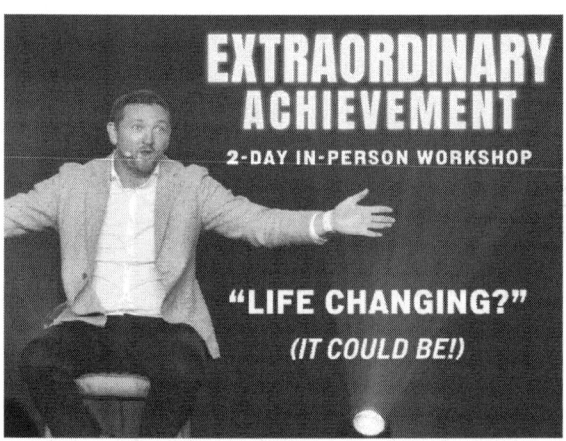

To Find Out When & Where In The World,
Register Your Interest At:

EXABook.com/Workshop

(Email: paul@paulgough.com)

Dedicated To Brendan Gough

This book is dedicated to all the people who told me I'd *never amount to anything*.

No it's not. Truth be told, there's not been that many. Other than my English teacher, who told my mother I wouldn't pass my English writing exam (the irony!), most people have been fairly supportive and encouraged me on my journey to entrepreneurial success.

None more so than my uncle **Brendan Gough** (pictured with me and my boys at a Hartlepool United soccer/football match).

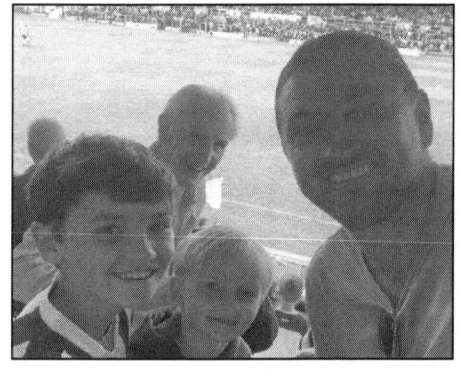

A few books ago (in *To Sell Is Healthy*) I mentioned my uncle Liam (Brendan's brother) and told you about the impact he's had on my life.

Well, this time I'd like to acknowledge Brendan. This guy has been one of my ultimate resources for advice on life and if my Uncle Liam instilled *belief* in me, then Brendan is the one who has constantly encouraged me to *enjoy my life* and make the most of it. Years later, now that I'm an adult doing adult things, he still finds time to check on how his "little nephew" is doing in life and ask if he needs anything.

This is the type of book I know Brendan has been reading for many years and I've read many suggested by him. His library is definitely bigger than his TV (more on that in Chapter 10).

Brendan, the thing I love about you most is *your love* for your family. Not just me, but *all* of us in it. It doesn't go unnoticed. I speak for all of your nephews and nieces when I say we talk about you a lot and everyone is in agreement that you are simply *the best*.

And **Brendan**, as much as many of the chats we had were in a nightclub, or at your kitchen table, and involved a fair amount of alcohol, I do remember most of them (I think!) and you've influenced me more than I could ever give you credit for. Thank you. My boys and I are lucky to have you in our lives ☺.

P.S And if you're a member of the family, wondering where *your* dedication is, hang on, I plan to write many more books. You will appear here soon.

Contents

Chapter Zero

My Backstory (Read This First.)

Part 1

Chapter 1

Could Everything You've Been Told About What It Takes To "Achieve" Be Wrong?

Chapter 2

Breaking Rules and Lovin' It!

Chapter 3

Ambition Creates Conflict

Chapter 4

What Drives You On Can Also Drive You Mad

Chapter 5

Why Is Everybody So Serious?

Part 2

Chapter 6

Five-Star Qualities

Chapter 7

Time Poverty

Chapter 8

Distractions Delay Progress

Chapter 9

Rough Diamonds

Chapter 10

The Hard Thing About Big Decisions

Part 3

Chapter 11

When They Zig, You Zag

Chapter 12

Balance Is Bullshit

Chapter 13

Approval Not Needed

Chapter 14

The Ultimate Investment

Chapter 15

The Unreasonable Club

Bonus Audio Chapters

Chapter 16

The 7 Habits of Hugely Successful Entrepreneurs

Chapter 17

What To Focus On Next: 6 Things That Should Get Your Time And Attention After This Book

Start Here

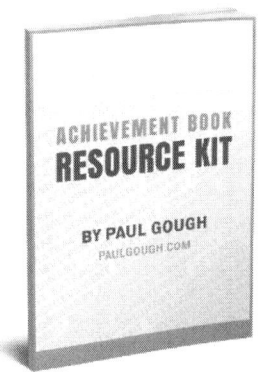

Get Your FREE Resources That Accompany The Extraordinary Achievement Book, Including:

✓ **The Self-Assessment Scorecard** - rate yourself on the principles discussed in this book and find out the areas in which you need to make improvements on to get to that next level of success faster.

✓ **The Checklist/Poster** - get a copy of all of the principles discussed in one place so you can print it out, put it on your wall and make each one easier to remember and implement into your life.

✓ **Instant Access Video** - Watch me talk about some of these principles **LIVE** on stage.

✓ **Bonus Audio (Chapter 16)** - The 7 Habits of Hugely Successful Entrepreneurs

✓ **Bonus Audio (Chapter 17)** - What to Focus On Next: 6 Things That Should Get Your Time And Attention After This Book

✓ **Free Chapters** - Get the first two chapters of my best-selling book Leadership In Private Practice.

✓ **Surprise Items** - Plus, at least two other surprise items that if you have enjoyed this book, I know you will love.

Go To This Page Now:
EXAbook.com/Free

ACHIEVEMENT
CHAPTER ZERO

Read This First
"Imagine A Life That Is Free From Guilt, Fear, And Regret..."

I know that most introductions like this are often skipped in favour of getting straight to the "meat" of the book. As much as I encourage and admire such eagerness to learn, such a thing will not be helpful in this situation. **This introduction *is* worth reading.**

Let's start by doing a little bit of "imagining" about a life that is available to you and perhaps waiting for you at the end of this book. Ready? Here goes:

- ✓ *Imagine* a life that is free from guilt, fear, and regret…
- ✓ *Imagine* a life where you could make loads of money and *not* regret what you had to do or give up getting it…

- ✓ *Imagine* for a second a life where you didn't have to worry what others think of you, and you didn't need their approval to do things that are important to you…
- ✓ *Imagine* a life where you figured out how to make loads of money and the reason you did so was because you gave up on the idea of *trying to do it all on your own*…
- ✓ *Imagine* a life where you stopped taking life so seriously and in fact found fun in just how seriously *everyone else* takes it…
- ✓ *Imagine* a life where you are comfortable making big decisions and even if you get one wrong, you are still happy…
- ✓ *Imagine* a life where you don't feel forced to follow outdated rules, where you accept yourself even if others question how you live…
- ✓ *Imagine* a life that, when faced with the choice of following the crowd or your own intuition, you have the courage to say "to hell with the crowd" and go your way…
- ✓ *Imagine* a life where you got wealthy and it didn't matter who the government is, or what agenda is being pushed, or by whom…
- ✓ *Imagine* being able to use time to your advantage to get more things done, so you make more money than you ever have, despite working less…
- ✓ *Imagine* you could discover what is really motivating you and finally understand why you're *still* unhappy or restless despite having experienced a good deal of success already…
- ✓ *Imagine* being able to defy your parents' life path for you—and being OK with it…

- ✓ Now *imagine* being able to look into the eyes of your kids and even though they say they "don't want you to go to work" because "they miss you," *you do so anyway*, guilt free, knowing for certain it's in everyone's best interest that you do…
- ✓ Then *imagine* waking up every day knowing that you will get done what you say you will and nothing will get in the way…
- ✓ And finally, *imagine* making so much money that your in-laws would be forgiven for thinking that you've won the lottery—or turned to drug dealing— and you don't care which one they think as you're too busy having fun spending it all…

Well….

Now look, I'm not promising you *all* of that will happen just by reading this book, but *I am* suggesting that is just some of what is *possible* by reading *Extraordinary Achievement*.

Sure, it's about success and achievement, making money, experiencing the finer things, and getting to the next level of life. **But it's really about finding a way to enjoy life and feel good about yourself as you live it.** That's the premise of the book and that's also the promise of this book.

It's about finding a way to make money and *enjoy* the process of doing so. It's about building a successful business, living with less guilt and less fear, as well as being OK with making big decisions that currently may scare you (Chapter 10).

It's about backing yourself, being certain in yourself, and living in a way that recognizes the only fix that needs to be made to who you are is accepting how good you already are (Chapter 3). It's a book about a better future that doesn't overlook today. It's a book about making money that doesn't lose sight of having fun and *not taking life too seriously* (Chapter 5).

It's a book that regularly pokes fun at some of the stupid ideals, false beliefs, and outdated ways of living that, in this author's opinion, are holding people back from enjoying a good life and should have been left in the 16th century, where most of them came from.

What is more, and perhaps most important, it's a book about balancing your **entrepreneurial ambition with acceptance of yourself**.

It's about wanting a bit more, getting a bit more, but *without* doing so at your own expense. And by "own expense" I mean how you feel about yourself in the process of getting it. It's about getting "it," whatever "it" is, without kicking yourself or putting yourself down on the way.

It's about being OK with what you've got right now, and how you feel about yourself right now, but still finding a way to achieve more. And not because you want more to feel better about yourself, or your life, but because growth and progress are at the very heart of who you are and what you're here for.

It's about using the insecurities you've got to drive you on, without driving you mad (the subject of Chapter 4.)

It's about finding a way to grow, to overcome challenges and obstacles that will allow you to look back and be proud of what you did, and how much you achieved, without regretting what you had to give up getting there (Chapter 11).

It's about making a lot of money, not because you think it'll make you feel safer or more secure, or any better than anyone else, but because you wanted to have more fun and experience more fun things in life. The type of things that only money can buy.

If you want any of that, you will love this book and I encourage you to read every word at least once.

Why Did I Write This Book?

So that's what it's all about. The next question I guess I need to answer in this introduction is *why I decided to write this book*.

As well as being a *lonely* entrepreneur, I'm also a fairly *busy* entrepreneur ("good busy") running four companies and raising just as many kids. I've got plenty to occupy my time and in between the kids and my companies I like to sit by my pool, enjoy the Florida sun, and sip margaritas.

So why on earth did I invest hundreds of hours—actually, over a thousand—in writing this book that, although worth hundreds of thousands of dollars in terms of the advice inside available to you, will sell for no more than a measly $35?

Believe me, there were many days and weekends where I questioned precisely why I did so. Especially when it was hot and sunny outside and I could have been lounging by said pool with said margarita in hand listening to Jimmy Buffett sing "It's Five O'Clock Somewhere."

Well, let me tell you, as I think it's important for you to know.

I wrote it because about ten years ago I discovered that what I was doing, how I was living, and how I was motivated to make money was *unhealthy*. I realized that unless I figured that out, and corrected it, it meant I was always going to be *unsettled*, *insecure*, *fearful* and *restless*—and no amount of money I made from my business would ever change that.

I didn't like the idea of having money but living my life with angst and always in the future, never happy or settled with what I had today, so I went away and figured out how to change it.

I want to share that discovery with you in the hope of helping *you* become more comfortable with who you are as well as raise or re-ignite your belief in yourself and *ideally* separate that from any business or monetary success that comes your way.

I believe personal security is more important than financial security and I say so because often when you get the former, soon after you get the latter.

Most people go their whole lives never realizing the reason they're lacking financially is because they're lacking in the place where it matters most—how they feel about themselves and the *belief* they have that they could never be anything *but* poor.

I wrote it because I see far too many entrepreneurs who are successful but unhappy. And that's got to be the ultimate failure. I believe it happens so frequently because too many are living to please others, always seeking *approval from others,* and in doing so are never really living a day of their own lives. They have "everything" but at the same time they have nothing but regret and frustration.

If you can't do what you want, with whom you want and even feel how you want, what have you got, I ask?

Autonomy is the key to a great life that you can call your own and it'll be discussed in depth in the coming pages.

So why else did I write it?

@THEPAULGOUGH

I wrote it to help people be happy with what they've got and who they are right now, without losing the *ambition* to want more.

The problem for many people is that they are always wanting more, always thinking that their lives will somehow be better when they've got more. But as many find out, they're nearly always left disappointed even when they get it. I want to share a different way as there's a solution other than always thinking you need more money and giving up your life to get it.

I wrote it to encourage more entrepreneurs to think bigger, pursue growth, enjoy more prosperity, and to be brazen about wanting to *make more money*, and do it in a way that allows you to enjoy the process of doing so.

I wrote it because I know there are millions of businesses owners who live every day feeling *judged, guilty,* and *fearful* of the future, and no matter what they do, or how much they make, none of it ever seems to go away.

I wrote it because I know that having a good bit of money allows you to experience the finer things in life. I'm talking about the things that without money you're limited to watching happen on TV or via the Instagram accounts of celebrities and sports stars.

I wrote it because I believe that entrepreneurs are the most *impactful* people in any society—jobs don't create themselves—and very few people give us the credit we deserve despite the risks we take and heartache we endure.

Moreover, I wrote it because I believe wholeheartedly in the human potential and I know that every single person reading this book is capable of more, no matter what level they're currently at. Sometimes, most times, all you need is the *permission* to do the thing you knew all along you should be doing.

GET YOUR ACHIEVEMENT BOOK RESOURCE KIT: WWW.EXABOOK.COM/FREE

In that way, this book is a 250+-page *permission slip* **that will grant everyone who dares cash it the** *go-ahead* **to finally enjoy life, feel good about it, and care** *less* **about what others think about that.**

And, ideally, become seriously loaded along the way!

Finally, I wrote this book to help everyone who's ever experienced the *hell*, the setbacks, the *pressure*, the constant *worry*, and never-ending *challenges* that come with running and growing a business in the hope that when you look back on your day, your week, your month, perhaps your life, you will be able to say that it was worth it and that, maybe, your only regret would be that you couldn't go and do it all again.

I want you to get to the end and say, "What a ride that was. Can I play again?"

Much better than getting to the end and asking, "Was that it?" or worse, saying "Thank goodness that's over!"

Finally, I have an understanding of precisely what entrepreneurs have to go through and after spending a **lot of my own time, money, and effort on figuring out to how enjoy life and make a good bit of money,** I wanted to share that in the hope of inspiring others to do the same.

You, I hope.

And Finally, "Who The Heck Is This Paul Gough Guy?"
Good Question. Here's My Back Story...

So that's what this book is *about*, *who* it's for, and *why* I wrote it. The final thing I'd like to share before you *rush off* to *devour* Chapter 1 is who I am and how I came to be in a position to write this in the first place.

What you're about to read is no ordinary book on achievement or success, so I think it's important you know **where** and **who** it comes from.

If you're going to read a book written in a way that is very likely to challenge your every belief about life and success, that will probably be in direct conflict with things you've been told by people you love, know, and trust, I think it's only fair to know a bit about the person you're going to hear from, before you hear from him.

We're strangers right now, and I'd like for you to get a *bit more comfortable* with me and my background so you can settle into the book without constantly wondering who the heck I am, or as is more likely, where the heck I got the *audacity* to say many of the things I am going to say in this book.

With that said, allow me to introduce myself.

My full name is *Paul Andrew Gough* and I was born in 1981. It means when I finished this book I was 42 years old. I'm from a small, somewhat economically challenged, town in the northeast of England called Hartlepool. I'm a very happy-go-lucky kind of guy, and although I often talk to hundreds of people at a time in my seminars, I'm more comfortable in a group of two or three at most and for that reason I mostly keep myself to myself.

I love to laugh and have fun and *I like to think* I am also very good-humored.

If you ask me where I live, I wouldn't tell you Florida, I'd tell you I live in a *playful state*.

@THEPAULGOUGH

I definitely don't take life seriously and I often break rules. In fact, I *love* breaking rules. It's one of my favorite things to do.

I love watching and playing soccer with my boys (Hartlepool United and Liverpool FC are my teams) and I have a love of margaritas developed since moving to Florida. It's always five o'clock somewhere in Orlando and if it isn't, it will be back in my home country of England, so I'm covered either way.

I've got four kids and apart from the occasional night out with a friend or two, I spend almost all of my spare time with my boys and Natalie, my wife. Just how I like it. Just how I chose it.

I'll spare you the first 18 years of my life except to say that I was raised by two fantastic parents, and I was given all the opportunities to live and enjoy my life that I could ever wish for. I think about that childhood *a lot* and I'm sure it plays a big part in my success today.

I have a large extended family, one side of it mostly of Irish heritage (my dad's), and I include my grandma and grandad in the enjoyment that I had growing up, not forgetting my sister, my brother, my cousins, aunties, and uncles, too numerous to mention. Family is important to me and I love to hang out with them *any* opportunity I get.

Things got *interesting* for me when I was about 18 and I decided not to follow in the career path my father had planned for me.

He will likely have a different opinion of it, but for me, that is the day that a lot of problems between me and my dad surfaced and also coincided with a time of my life where I was feeling a *lot* insecure. There's more on this in Chapter 4, but this period of time definitely had a big impact on my life. More than I knew at the time.

Anyway, at 19, I went off to university in a place called Newcastle, a cool city in the UK, and I did a degree in physiotherapy. I'd have loved to play professional soccer, but I wasn't good enough and decided that being a physiotherapist would allow me to stay around sport.

And I was right. It did.

I landed my first job as a physiotherapist working for a small team called Darlington FC and soon after that I started working with a big team called Middlesbrough FC, who were in the English Premier League at the time.

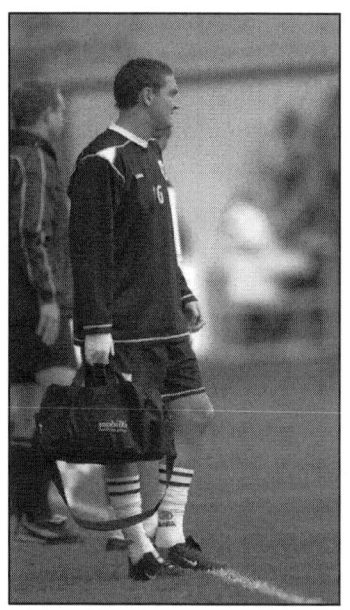 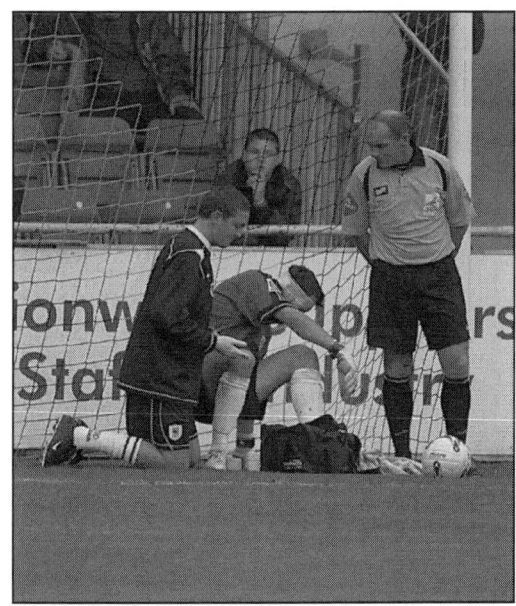

(That's me in my early career attending to an injured soccer/football player.)

After a few years of working in professional soccer, I realized I didn't love it as much as I did at the start, so I left to pursue my own career in private practice.

@THEPAULGOUGH

I went and started my own company, The Paul Gough Physio Rooms, in 2008 and in less than twelve years that "small" little physio business, on the corner of a small town in the northeast of England, that I started from scratch, with zero money, no business skills, and nothing but hope and a bit of enthusiasm, got to four locations, provided 50 people with good jobs, and has generated well over $10,000,000 in mostly cash pay revenue, in a country with a completely free socialist health care system as my main competitor (the National Health Service).

The *Paul Gough Physio Rooms* has done so well over the years that its name and reputation, its brand, is about to be licensed to other physical therapists to allow its impact to reach even further. I have no regrets in quitting my day job in soccer, nor do I have any regrets about what happened next…

On the back of the success of that business, I started another one called *Paul Gough Media.*

This company works primarily with physical therapy and other private practice owners in the USA, UK, Ireland, Canada, Australia, and New Zealand—and as far away as Bahrain and Thailand—and we sort out their marketing and help them scale without needing doctors. Many even come to us for advice on how to escape the rabbit hole (death trap!) that is the insurance reimbursement system.

I also created *PhysioFunnels*—the software technology that powers the marketing automation of many very successful private practices around the world (www.physiofunnels.com).

Most of my clients at the start were from the USA, so that meant my family and I "had" to move to Orlando to make it work. We're conveniently located just five minutes from Disney World and it is sunny 300+ days of the year. The taxes are good here as well.

It was a hard decision.

I run seminars all over the world, from London to Las Vegas, Dublin, and Sydney, and I've written five other best-selling books (www.paulgoughbooks.com).

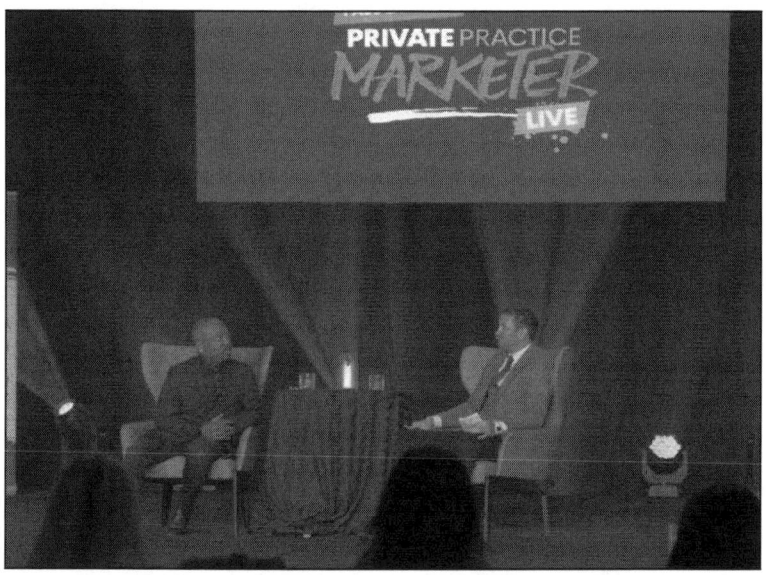

(That's me on stage with Daymond John, founder of FUBU and star of ABC's Shark Tank at one of my events, Private Practice Marker Live, that happens every year in Orlando)

My podcast (The Paul Gough Podcast and Audio Experience) is on iTunes and at the time of publishing it's had more than *one million* plays.

I've generated millions and millions of dollars in revenue in the UK and the USA, hired people in both countries (and fired a few too!), and I've since built a property empire of more than 70 homes with zero debt.

@THEPAULGOUGH

I don't like banks. I can't stand their rules, so I decided to *become my own*.

These days I employ 40+ people between the UK and the USA, and I live between both. Winter in the USA, summer in the UK. I live in shorts. The only thing I really worry about is a bit of cloud in the UK, and hurricanes and mosquitos in Florida.

Most people can't work out what I do anymore, and that never fails to make me laugh.

All they know is I seem to have a nice life, I go all over the world with my kids regularly, and if you pushed me, I think most would think I am a drug dealer, or I've won the lottery (neither are true, by the way).

I'm a self-made multi-millionaire and I've made every penny through building and operating businesses. It wasn't inherited, given, or won. It was *earned*.

I'm not the world's best business owner, but I am up there with how much I love being a business owner. It's a privilege to me, as is the pressure, and I never take it for granted. I'm obsessed with learning how business works and getting better at running one, and just how much often shows up on my tax return.

I have four children (*Harry, Tobias, Grayson, and Zander*), and an amazing partner in Natalie, who loves, supports, and wants me to be happy more than I could ever wish for. She's amazing. Individually we are great, put together we are better, and we have more fun in life than I could ever write and tell you.

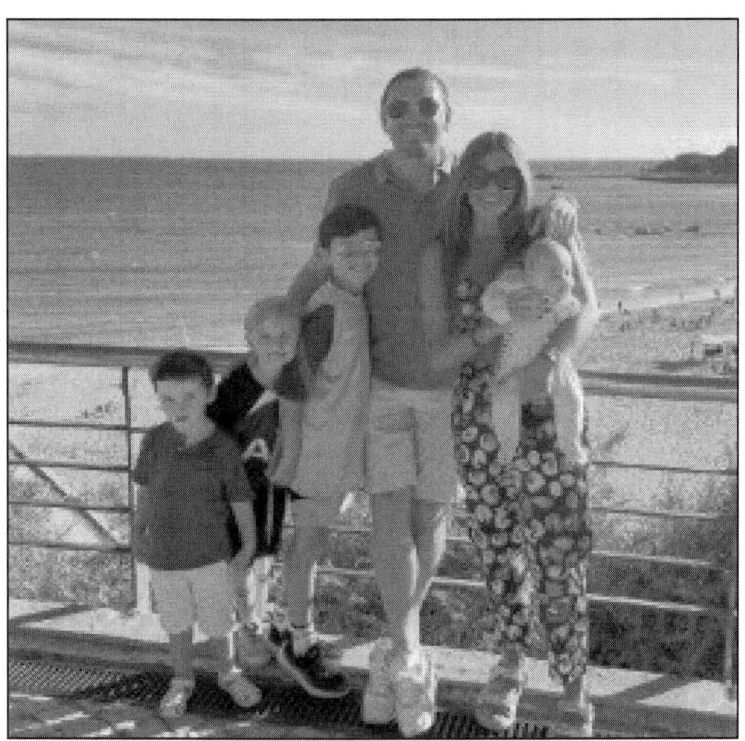

(That's us on vacation in our favorite place, Albufeira, Portugal. From left to right: Grayson, Tobias, Harry, me, Natalie, and Zander.)

I've done a lot, made a lot, and I've learned a lot. I've also made a few mistakes. Scrap that, I've made a *lot* of mistakes and I live my life knowing that how I've chosen to live it requires that I make a few more.

I share most of my experiences (business and life) in my books or at my seminars—sometimes to the dislike of many ex-staff—but that's the life I've chosen. I've learned that when I say things, so as long as it's not aimed at them, people seem love my ideas, my candid style and my different way of thinking. It's "refreshing."

However, the minute whatever I say involves questioning how they behave or act, all of a sudden I am the devil and everyone will hear about it or they will quit.

Anyway, I'm not your typical business owner stuck in an office, chained to the desk, never able to leave it, nor am I one of those business *theorists* turned business authors who like to sit behind a keyboard telling *real* business owners how to run a business, never having run one themselves.

I started my business in 2008, the year of the banking crisis, and I took on the challenge that was COVID and came out the other side with an even bigger, better, and stronger company. I've risked my own time and money to get to this point in life and everything has been earned and learned.

I've also had my heart broken on numerous occasions by dishonest staff and I've lost lots of money to great ideas I was sure were going to be winners.

Despite the success of the business, and putting my family aside, I'd say my biggest achievement in life is that I figured out and faced up to a few insecurities that, if I hadn't, would have meant all of the "success" that I've had commercially would have been diluted and hard to enjoy.

When I was about 30 (ish), I had a feeling that something wasn't right, despite making so much money. I had a feeling that even though my bank balance was doing well, I had a Porsche 911 on the drive and a big house all to myself, there was something not quite right in how I felt about myself and how I was living.

I set off on a bit of a journey to discover what that was, and I learned a good many things on the way. Many of those things I am sharing in this book. They are *not* right or wrong, good or bad, they are simply things that have worked for me to help me get to the point I am today. That is more secure, less restless, having more fun, and with a bit more money at my disposal than I realistically will ever need.

If you want any or all of those, there's no doubt you will love this book, and it will have been worth reading to discover how I got them.

As we go through this book together, remember that I *will* challenge many of your existing beliefs about success and how money is made, even the role that others have played in your life and question if it's time to fire a few from it.

The promise on the front of the book is *big* and *bold* and it requires some big, bold statements as well as the confrontation of many out dated "truths." It won't always be an easy read. I will say things you won't agree with (yet) and I *will* make you uncomfortable from time to time.

Finally, as you will discover throughout the book, I am nothing if not upfront, honest, and candid. British people are often tolerant, compliant, and love to *keep calm and carry on regardless*. All great traits to have, but sadly, I do not possess any of them.

Which brings me nicely to the next and final section of this introduction.

If You Are Easily Offended...

As you may or may not pick up on during this book, I have a writing style, and a sense of humor, that is not typical of a "professional" author under contract with a "professional" publisher.

(It is a good thing I am neither then, isn't it?)

It's why, despite many lucrative offers from many reputable publishing companies, I prefer to publish my own books. Doing so means I can say pretty much what I want and do not have to take something out that perhaps the publishing people do not agree with, fail to understand, or think might offend someone.

And that's the real big difference between me and these professional publishing people.

See, their goal is to make sure that *no one* is offended.

My goal is to at least *try* to do so.

In the coming pages of this book, I will make a point of openly mocking many of the *senseless* things that seem to occur so frequently in society, that often go unquestioned, and make no hiding of the fact that I'm *occasionally* doing so for my own amusement.

Ninety thousand words is a lot of hours and I have to get some entertainment from somewhere. I often do it through my writing. That said, just because I am having so much fun, that should not distract you from the *seriousness* with which I present to you some of the *thoughtless* stuff that is going on around you, that should not be copied and at the very least needs questioning.

Rest assured, if you are easily offended, and *get off* on such a thing, then you will probably love this book and it possibly will make your day. There'll be something in every chapter that will trigger you and you won't have to look that hard to find it. If you are in the mood to be offended, then this book is your ticket to being so.

There. You have been forewarned and, equally, I have made my promise.

@THEPAULGOUGH

Let's Get Started

OK, with all that said, first get your free resources that accompany this book at: **WWW.EXABOOK.COM/FREE** then get your highlighter ready to mark important parts that you wish to come back to later, remove the top, put it in your other hand, and let's get into the "meat" of the book.

I've broken the book into three parts. There are 15 chapters in total, and the first one starts with a look at why so many people are so unhappy in the entrepreneurial world, despite having achieved so much. Let's go!

PART 1

ACHIEVEMENT
CHAPTER 1

Could Everything You've Been Told About What It Takes To "Achieve" Be Wrong?

One of the biggest challenges for any entrepreneur is finding the balance between growing a successful business, attempting to make lots of money from that business, and being able to say that you enjoyed both the process of doing so—*and* your life. What an Achievement that would be if you could say you did it.

Would you agree?

Although desirable, such a life is no easy task. Millions of entrepreneurs have tried and failed at figuring out a method for building a successful business and simultaneously enjoying a terrific life.

For a small minority, it is a successful business at the *expense* of a terrific life; it is a lot of money but a life of struggle and stress.

And sadly, for the overwhelming majority, it is a quadruple whammy of a *bad* business with lots of hassle, mountains of debt, and, worst of all, a life plagued by guilt over missing out on so much family time trying to make it work.

With all that said, surely it's not just me thinking, "What's the point of either?" (And yes, even the money?)

Seriously, what's the point of having a load of money if you're too unhealthy to enjoy it, don't know how to enjoy it, or dare not enjoy it for fear of running out of it?

And what's the point of building a successful business that makes lots of money if you're perpetually stressed and miserable because of what you must do to make it all? Or, just as bad, worried about what people think of you now that you're successful and find yourself with more money available to you than most other people you know?

Doing the same thing every day and expecting a different result is the definition of insanity. So is *self-imposed* misery. And business owners have a wonderful knack of inflicting it upon themselves on a daily basis.

See, there's this belief in the entrepreneurial world that business *has* to be a grind, that it *has* to be tough, that you *have* to work crazy hours and you *have* to give up the best parts of your life to make it work. The theory is that if you do all of that, and if you persevere long enough, then "one day," "someday," it will all finally come together, and you can say you "did it".

I don't know about you, but to me, all that sounds like a lot to go through for just "one day" that might happen "someday."

Now such a thing might be *common* in the business world, but it should never be considered *normal*. And nor should it ever be a way of living you think *you* have to endure—just because everyone else does.

No amount of money will ever make up for three decades of stress, worry, not seeing kids and living your life like this "one day" will make up for everything you had to endure on the way to getting there. Only people who didn't figure out a better way will tell you otherwise. Or, those who get a kick out of moaning about their self-imposed misery. And there *are* such people out there. Lots of them. Just look on Facebook for proof.

But let me make something very clear from the start: this is not some *holier-than-thou* book about money being the "root of all evil". It's not one that tells you to give up on your ambition and be happy with what you've got, and it's definitely not about telling you that you're somehow greedy if you want more—however much you have.

I'll say right away that I believe it's great to have loads of money.

And even if you have enough to fill up a swimming pool, there's nothing wrong with wanting a bit more to jump into. We each have different aspirations and life goals for what we might need that money for. Just because someone judging you doesn't share those goals—or doesn't have goals as lofty—doesn't mean you're wrong and they're right.

Besides, you can do a lot of good for a lot of people, as well as have a lot of fun in your own life, once you get past the amount you need for day-to-day survival.

If in doubt, fill the pool with a bit more of it anyway. There'll never be a time where having more won't come in handy. Just be mindful of what you must give up getting it and make sure it's worth it. Keep one eye on your ambition, the other on being content with who you are and how you feel about yourself and you're going to have a terrific life.

@THEPAULGOUGH

What I find interesting about the pursuit of money is just how many people say they're *not* interested in it, and yet there they are lining up to play the Lottery every week, to get a bit more of it.

It's been my observation that it's usually the same people spouting that "Money is the root of all evil" or "The rich are all greedy," who are the first ones in line waiting to put their numbers on for this week's draw. Especially if it's a double roll over and the jackpot is five million instead of two million.

Here's the first big lesson in the book: the world is full of people who have figured out how to manipulate any situation to suit their view of the world, at any time they like. If there's a subject that people have become world class at these days, it is self-validation without any consideration of someone else's point of view.

They can line up to play the lottery because their "need" to win a few million dollars is justifiable, and needed, but *your* pursuit of it, well, that is just corporate greed and another example of how the world is unfair.

More on this Chapter 4, but for now, if you ever had the feeling that the world is full of self-righteous hypocrites, manipulating every situation to suit their *current* worldly view (and uphold their *own* lofty self-image), then your intuition would be correct and in pursuit of a terrific life, you will need to learn to navigate through and around such absurdity.

Make no mistake, money absolutely is important in this life. It simply has to be factored into the conversation about enjoying it a bit more. Being *on* the safari is much better than *watching* someone else do it on TV.

Despite most people's thinking there *is*, there's really *no* great mystery to getting your hands on plenty of it. And to make it even easier, the rules of how it flows have never changed in hundreds of years.

In business, money is collected as the reward for solving other people's problems. The bigger the problem, the more you make. That's it! That's the basic premise of running a business and how you get paid. Just solve people's problems and bill them for the opportunity of doing so.

It means if you keep solving their problems, they'll keep giving you money, and if you do that for long enough, you'll probably end up with more than you need. Control your spending habits, invest wisely, and there's an inevitability to one day becoming very rich. It's a really simple system and there's nothing mysterious or magical about it. Only it's stunning simplicity.

Sure, it relies upon a bit of imagination and creativity—as well as effort and intention applied to a commercial entity called a business—but those are things that are *easily* available to all. None of those things are being kept hidden, locked away in the Tower of London where only the lucky few can get in. They're available to every person, at any time, and best of all they're genuinely one of the few things in life that are free.

It's why I say there's nothing evil or greedy about wanting, getting or having a bit of cash. All there ever is, and ever has been, is a lack of understanding about how the system really works. And as you will discover in later chapters, the system really isn't designed with your prosperity in mind. In fact, it's not even designed with you in mind at all.

Money Is Misunderstood

Money is a contentious subject. It's hugely misunderstood. The bigger problem is that society has been conditioned to think that the way to *guarantee* a great life is to have loads of it. It's assumed that when you have enough then your every worry will disappear, and eternal happiness is granted to you.

It's why people without money generally think the answer to all of life's problems is to make more money. And equally, it's why the people who've already got loads of it think the answer to all *their* life's worries is to make more as well.

But whether you have no money and think getting some will sort everything *or* you've already got loads and think you need a top-up, surely someone must be wrong?

If you think you need more money to feel assured about yourself when you've got zero in the bank—and equally, if you think you need more money to feel assured when you've got a million large in the bank—there's got to be something else going on, right?

Well, *there is*.

And this, I believe, is the real problem—especially for entrepreneurs.

We quickly connect making more money from the business with feeling better about ourselves. We quickly connect a successful business with being a successful businessperson. And we quickly connect being a successful businessperson with being a great husband, wife, partner, parent, or friend.

If we're not careful, all our self-worth is tied to the success of the business and the only way to measure that is in the amount of money it makes.

It feels great when we have some—but what about when we have a bad month of sales, or an unexpected tax bill comes in? It happens. And when it does, how do you feel if all your personal worth is indexed against the amount in your bank and then when you look, all you see is red?

I don't need you to tell me—I already know.

You feel insecure, vulnerable, and a failure. The same as I *used* to.

Most of us are conditioned to believe that there's no safety without the security of a good personal economy. We can accept the thought of other things going wrong—such as our relationships and even health—but there's *real* fear in having no money. You need money to survive in this life and without it your only options are to beg, rob a bank, or steal from the local 7-11 in order to eat and stay alive. None are desirable options for most of us.

But here's the thing: despite what society will think, most people's biggest problem is not a lack of money. No. It is the belief that other people think *badly of them and how they feel about that.* That's right, the real problem most people live with is the idea that other people see them in a negative way. Business owners included.

Most people don't just want to *feel better*. They want to feel better *about themselves,* and it's assumed that with more money that will happen instantly.

Sure, with more money you can buy a luxury car and a bigger house or get new, whiter teeth, fuller lips, and an expensive suit to change someone's perceptions of you.

And all of these things are great, in and of themselves. Especially if you have a front tooth missing. But these are all *external* things that distract from the *internal* negativity people have about themselves.

What I am saying is all of these fancy things are great to have, but they don't do too much to fix a lack of self-belief, which, is most people's *real* problem in life.

That's why if you think *all* you need is a bit more money and *all* of your problems will go away, then you're in for a big shock. There's a reason millionaires hang themselves and rock stars continually overdose and it's not because they don't have enough cash, cars, or expensive watches. There's obviously something else going on.

It's why I ask the question at the outset of this chapter: "Could everything you've been told about achievement be wrong?"

As entrepreneurs, we mostly judge how much we've achieved in the last twelve months simply by looking at how much money we've made. It's a very simple system that has gone unchallenged for years and on the face of it, makes perfect sense. After all, you're in business to make money.

But it doesn't tell the whole story. As you're about to find out, there's a lot more to living an *extraordinary* life than just the pursuit of money. Being married is one thing. But being *happily* married is another. And equally, being rich is one thing. But being *happily* rich is another.

Should money be discounted as something you need to live a terrific life? Absolutely *not*.

It is vital. It is a prerequisite to being able to enjoy the finer things in life that only having money will allow you to do. As I write this chapter, I am sitting in the first-class cabin of a Virgin Atlantic flight from England to the USA. A quick look down the aisle and seeing 250+ passengers rammed in like a tin of sardines in economy reminds me that it is a lot more fun where I am. It also cost me an extra $7,500 to do it.

There's Nothing Bad About Wanting More Money

So, money really does make you a bit happier. And who ever said it doesn't probably never had any or is sitting in a cave somewhere singing a hymn or two on their homemade banjo oblivious to the commercial needs of life.

Money absolutely *does* have a place in your life and there's nothing evil about it at all.

Sure, there are a few dumb politicians who think so and would like to see all wealth re-distributed "evenly." But like I say, they're just dumb. They don't realize that even if all the money in the world *was* redistributed evenly and equally, it would only be a matter of time before it found its way back to the people the politicians stole it from in the first place.

Unbeknownst to politicians, money pays more attention to things like a strong work ethic, controlled spending habits, and high personal standards than any Robin Hood-style redistribution of it, however much they wish it were not true. It's why I believe the best thing politicians can ever do is not have people believe that the rich are evil—it would be to highlight how they got rich in the first place.

Start by reminding people that going to work is good, actually working when you are there is even better, and point out that when you've done that, you've earned the right to come home at night feeling proud of the commitment you made to *yourself*. This is a much better feeling than any drug or alcohol that you could ever buy, or, receiving a handout from the state that you really didn't need.

Wishful thinking, I know, but I'm sure glad that I found that way of living early in my life.

Besides, if you're into "conscious capitalism" or "fixing humanity" through your business, and other good stuff like that, you can *use your loot* to help out others, any time you like. You don't need to wait for shady politicians to redistribute it *from* you.

It's as simple as whenever you've made a bit too much money from your business, commit to spending lots of it! Do your bit for humanity (and the economy) by *spending* a good chunk of the dough you make and in doing so help other businesses make more money and create more good jobs for other people.

And, have a lot of fun doing so, of course.

If ever there was *a* single reason to get rich, I would argue it is to free yourself from the day-to-day mental torture of constantly living to survive. There's just something about money—or a lack of it—that does crazy things to your ability to focus on the small things that are really important to you.

Many marriages end because of disputes over its absence and it's almost impossible to notice your kids growing up if you're always worried about the next rent payment being due.

All of this considered, I believe that wanting more money isn't necessarily a bad thing and why you should do everything legally possible to get a bit more of it.

Having a bit more than you need to live, at the very least, gives you a chance to get your head above worry and start to notice important things in life that are currently passing you by. Plus, with more money, you can have a better education and top-class medical care. And things like that are vitally important to a great quality of life.

And besides, let's not sugar coat this, a $200 bottle of Champagne tastes much nicer than a $20 bottle, flying first class is much better than economy, and luxury houses, cars, and private chefs are definitely not just for movie stars or elite athletes. They're waiting for anyone with the courage to go get them.

(You, I hope?)

And by the way, living this way is not a sign that you're now "above yourself" or a sign that you've forgotten where you've come from or anything else that your parents or friends might want to throw at you. Far from it, actually.

What these things really mean is that you did something a little different than the people who *assume* they can't have those things. That's it!

It shows that you were *not* willing to accept the status quo and despite the fact you didn't come from a family where luxury was inherited, or wealth granted upon you, and even though your family might have told you that all rich people are "nasty" (more on that later), you decided to give it a go anyway and find out for yourself what all the fuss is about at the next level of life and comfort.

Really, they're all signs that you were prepared to make a few mistakes in pursuit of your ambition when the people around you made the biggest mistake of all—giving up on it.

Whatever they say, or you think they're saying, what *I'm* saying is there should be zero guilt on your part about any pursuit of money, comfort, better choices, or luxuries in your life. None whatsoever. You are simply *having a go* at achieving a quality to your life that others lack the ambition to ever make possible.

Ambition, the desire to raise yourself past the level where you currently are, is one of the most powerful driving forces in life. It's a word that will come up many times in this book. It is an important trait for an entrepreneur to have and it should never be dampened—not by anyone. Especially not your family or those *rat-bag* politicians who love to guilt anyone who is successful into feeling like they're to blame for everyone else's poverty and misery.

If in doubt, remember that you can't help them if you're one of them. The best thing you can do for poor people is to agree to *not* be one of them. Don't burden the system any more than it already is.

Whatever you achieve and wherever you land, it doesn't mean that you must forget your roots, nor does it mean you've gotten above yourself if you make it to the "big time." Whatever that even means. No. It just means you have a level of *curiosity* that the people in your family who went before you, obviously didn't. You could see something they couldn't, and you had the courage to go after it and get it.

Well done to you! You deserve everything you get and I for one would celebrate with you for doing so.

Can We Agree on This Idea?

Now with all that said, we're at an important junction in the book. If the rest of what you're going to read is to be *relevant* and *useable*, we need to agree early on in this book that having a lot of money is pretty cool—and definitely more desirable than not. But, we must also acknowledge that it's not a cure for many of the problems that entrepreneurs like you and I face.

Living with insecurity and doubt, feeling a little lost and lonely, as well as spending your every moment trying to work out how to make the future better than the past, are just some of the problems we face each day and yet, sadly, all of the money in the world won't fix any of them.

It's why the pursuit of money in and of itself is a fool's game. Especially if you think having loads is going to rid you of any those things I've just mentioned.

It's why I believe the real journey that you're on is to find a way to *balance your ambition* with that of complete acceptance of yourself and who you are. It's cool to want a bit more, but not if you think it makes you somehow *better* for getting it.

Which brings me to *why* I wanted to write this book.

The book is about sharing a method for making loads of money and at the same time, **enjoying life and feeling good about yourself as you live it.**

Which sounds nice, right?

It's about living more securely, with less doubt and feeling more confident about yourself so that even though you *could* go and buy that brand new Bentley Continental soft top, for cash, it wouldn't change anything in terms of how you feel about yourself if you did.

For you, buying it such a car would be nothing more than an acknowledgment of the commercial progress you've made, or, a dream being realized. And oh yes, maybe a nice big "*F-U*" to anyone who told you not to start the business in the first place or doubted that you could make it work. Not that it should make *that* much difference to the quality of your life, but it's always nice to prove a couple of people wrong, right?

To be clear, what we're going to focus on in this book is how to feel great about yourself, how to become more secure in yourself, and through the process of doing so discover that money and the commercial success you crave becomes much easier to come by. So easy that it'll feel like the system is finally working for you and not against you.

"Ordinary with Extras": A Life Available to Everyone

This is a book about living Extraordinarily. It's about getting to the next level of life and living in a way that most others don't even know is possible.

Throughout, I'll be sharing with you many different principles and ways for living that I believe will help you live at the next level whether in business or life.

Principles, that I might add, have helped me to stockpile a few million dollars, and more, and with it, just as many laughs, memories, and enjoyable experiences. Not forgetting, feeling a lot more secure in myself as I go about living my life. The latter being *easily* the best reward of all.

Let's start by considering the following question: what does it really take to be, or live Extraordinary?

Well, it's simple, to be honest. Just be *ordinary*, with a few *extras*!

I'll say it again: Extraordinary is nothing but "ordinary" with "extras."

It's nothing magical, nothing special, and certainly nothing elusive to anyone reading this book. It is likely to be something you're already doing, or how you're already living, with one or two things added. In some cases, it could even be one or two things *removed*.

You might be pleased to know it is not more hard work, it's not more hustle, and it's definitely not more sacrifice. It's simply changing one or two things in the way that you live, how you think, and how you pursue success.

It might even involve breaking a few silly rules that someone you've never met created and it might mean irritating a few people as you do. Which is always fun. Especially if it's people who you've so far been forced to be nice to through gritted teeth or moral obligation. Like your parents, for example. Or, maybe even your partner?

If you could confidently say right now that you are living "ordinary"—and doing it well—then you're already 80 percent of the way to living *Extra*ordinary. And yes, you will find the remaining 20 percent of what you need inside this book.

To get you moving in the right direction, one of the first things we must clarify is the difference between Achievement and success.

The two are very similar in that they both, in a roundabout way, cover the accomplishment of a goal or target. I could have easily called this book *Extraordinary Success* and it would have been appropriate. However, Achievement, in my eyes, is something that transcends success. Achievement sits atop success.

And here's why: in the simplest view, success is getting what you want from life or business. It's often about *getting* something, *owning* something, *becoming* someone, or even *proving* something to someone else. And at various points in their lives, all entrepreneurs are motivated in some way by one of those things. Sometimes, it's all of them all at once.

Success is nice, but Achievement, well, that is something else altogether.

Achievement is more about *how* you got it and how you *feel* about it as well as how long it lasts. It is the emotional aspect of success.

I firmly believe the point of life is to *enjoy it and feel good about yourself as you live it.* That's why, in my eyes, and for the purpose of this book, Achievement trumps success because it factors in your happiness *and* fulfillment. It's the thing you *really* wanted or thought you would get from having the money or a successful business in the first place.

Achievement is getting what you want, feeling amazing about it, and *still* feeling that way many months later.

Achievement is the ability to get what you want and look back and say that you loved the journey you took. If you look back and there's lots of regret about what you had to do to get it, how much you had to sacrifice, or, worse, who suffered along the way, I'm not sure anything has been achieved. It's probably more accurate to say that more was given up than was ever gained.

If in doubt, remember that success without fulfilment is regarded the ultimate failure. If what you're doing or even getting *isn't* making you happier, more secure and allowing you to live with more self-belief, then you're on the wrong path and it needs addressing fast.

As I alluded to earlier, I believe the hardest task on your hands as an entrepreneur is to be able to hit your targets—financial included—without compromising anything that is of real value to you. And anything that is of real value is something that can't be bought.

If you must wear it, buy it, or own it to feel better about yourself, it probably isn't of real and lasting value and it's the wrong goal to focus on *if* you're looking change *how you feel* in the long term.

That's why you can't just focus on more money hoping when you've got enough, you'll suddenly feel better. You won't. You will just be more annoyed that despite having made more money you *still* don't feel good about yourself.

The trick is live in a way that focuses on your personal security first. It's to fix how you feel about yourself *first* and with that accomplished more often than not what happens is the financial security follows soon after.

We will discuss more on this later in the book, but basically, most people do it the other way—focus on finance first—and in doing so hope that their insecurities and vulnerabilities will disappear because of few extra zeros in the bank.

But as many find out, it doesn't work like that.

It's why in any conversation about success, you can't just look at your tax return to see how much money you made last year and decide if you're doing well.

In order to be a *well-rounded* individual, who happens to be *loaded*, you've also got to consider how your internal game is progressing as well. In the same twelve-month period of making seven figures profit, are you getting more or less secure in yourself? And, are you getting more confident in situations that in the past you may have felt uncomfortable in? If you are, you're making progress.

Another clue is how you feel about the decisions you made in the past. If the decisions you had to make a couple of years ago don't today seem much smaller and easier, almost trivial, then you're probably *not* making the type of progress you assumed would come as a result of the money.

As for self-assurance, if you still worrying over what other people think about you or what is expected of you, you're missing the point of the journey that you're on. You may be richer, but you're still poor in the place that matters most—your self-esteem.

Make no mistake, it is possible to make more money but not make progress with how you feel about yourself or how much you enjoy life.

However, if you are making progress with your self-belief, your ability to regulate how you feel about yourself independent of what anyone else thinks, and the problems you've got today are better ones than a year ago, then you're on the right track and *even if you're not* making as much money as you'd like, just stay the course, it won't be that long before the money shows up.

The Big Tax Bill Doesn't Tell The Full Story

To get both of these aspects of success right— the internal feeling of security and the big tax return—is possible. It's also vital. That's why over the last few years of my own entrepreneurial journey I've become obsessed with figuring out a way to grow my businesses, make more money, and provide a better lifestyle for my family—having nice things and experiencing the finer things in life—but doing it in a way that means I don't have to compromise or sacrifice the most important parts of myself. The things that *really* matter to me.

Things such as staying calm and focused when others are panicked or distracted, being consistent when others are erratic, and demanding just as much from myself as I do from others, have become more valuable to me that anything I own.

I've also learned to stay true to my character and what I know to be true about myself, as well as how to get what I want from life—even though everyone else assumes that is a selfish way of living.

What is more, I've discovered the value of being predictable and consistent with my emotions on a daily basis. Good people don't hang around with people who are volatile and wildly emotional. To be a successful entrepreneur you need good people around you. It means you must learn to control how you feel no matter how much stupid stuff goes on around you, and even if life seems to be conspiring against you.

Which it often can, especially when you start to hire lots of staff or a new strain of a virus makes its way around the world, shutting most of it for a year or two.

Admittedly, this way of living is not for everyone. It's not easy. You must live and think in a way that is mostly opposite from everyone else around you. And that can be uncomfortable to do so. Being in a pack and following along with the general or "popular" thinking about life is easy. It feels safe. But if you want to live differently—Extraordinarily—then you have to be OK with acting differently.

And that is made easier if you have a ferocious and unshakeable belief in yourself.

Self-belief is the secret sauce to a life with more progress and less fear, not to mention more things accomplished. Once you get it (covered more in Chapter 3), and you sprinkle on top a little shall we say "commercial savviness" (business skills), it's almost certain that the cash begins to flow in your direction and the only challenge you'll have is where to put it all.

What is more, I also believe that when you've figured it out for yourself, you should pass the instructions on to someone else. Show them how to do the same.

Far from being selfish, focusing on *yourself first* is about having the courage to accept that you can't help others unless you've first helped yourself. That's the bit people misunderstood about living *self first*. It's to do so with the pure intention of being able to help others.

Have I cracked it? Of course not. A work in progress? Absolutely!

I've come to accept and secretly love knowing that I'm always working on some part of myself that is out of sync. Finding "balance" is going to be a fight I will never win (as you will see in Chapter 11, "Balance is Bullshit"). But in making progress in all of the areas we'll cover in this book, I'll land a lot closer to the type of life that makes my life worth living and is not one saddled with fear and regret.

This may come as a shock, but life isn't about existing or surviving. Far from it.

It's about setting ambitious goals, dreaming big and enjoying it by making progress on realizing those dreams and feeling amazing about yourself as you do. It's about feeling alive, not just being alive. And it absolutely is about making enough money to thrive, not just survive.

I believe that is *real Achievement* in this life.

I also believe that *you* can do it too.

To many people in society, that type of life might seem unachievable or at least very unlikely. It might also sound a little greedy.

And maybe they are right?

But with that view of life, I ask, why would you even want to be right? Why would you bother getting out of bed if you really do believe that life must be a struggle, that you have to be poor, and that only lucky people end up rich?

Sounds like the view of someone who has already given up on life, if you ask me, and I assume that in picking up this book you want better for yourself than that.

If you do, you're going to love this book.

Throughout, you'll notice that I move between writing to you about ways to speed up success—offering practical tips to make you more productive, leverage other people's time and skills, build teams, make big decisions, and develop your focus, etc.—and how to hone the skills you'll need to enjoy the happy by-products of all of doing those things well: that being *more time, more money and more opportunity*.

Who knows, you may even find that as a result of everything you read in this book you will have more fun, smile more, and laugh more than you ever have before. Which will mean better and deeper relationships with the people on the journey with you.

It is a big, bold, promise, but if you're open-minded and willing to be challenged—just a little—I believe you can at least make a step or two in the right direction. Which would be nice, right?

Ready to get started? If so, let's move on to the next chapter together and get into my favourite subject—rule breaking!

Major Principle of Chapter 1: Money might make you happy, but it won't fix your insecurity problems. However, fixing your insecurity problems will probably make you a lot of money.

ACHIEVEMENT
CHAPTER 2

Breaking Rules And Lovin' It!

What do people with frustratingly average lives, with frustratingly average incomes, all have in common? One word: conformity.

That is, they all conform to *silly little rules* and outdated ways of living that keep people stuck at average. Think about it, if everyone follows the same rules, and lives and thinks the same way because of those rules, then by definition all those people become the sum of all that same activity. Somewhere in all this rule following is a whole lot of people stuck at average.

It's why many people, despite having a different life in *theory*, in reality, have the same sort of life as most of the people around them.

And there's nothing bad with any of it, I might add.

Except, that is, if you're looking to live extraordinarily.

Almost all of the success that you see anyone having that you admire has its roots in breaking rules. They refused to follow along with the crowd. They opted *out* of what you might call "popular delusion." That being a way of living that although embraced by many, makes no sense whatsoever and doesn't come up with the goods.

See, it's *not* the conformists who get what they want in this life.

And it's definitely not the timid.

It's the ones with the biggest "brass balls." That being a rather eloquent phrase we use in Britain that stands for courage and guts. Despite popular belief —or delusion perhaps?—the ones who get the life they really want are the ones with the courage to think and act differently and in doing so, get what most others don't.

It's not about copying what everyone around you is doing. It's about living beyond the *limitations of imitation.* Meaning, most of the limits you're experiencing in life happen because you're copying what others do who *also* have the same limitation in their life (as the one you're trying to avoid.) It's not how we're taught in school, but it is how it works in the world of achievement.

See, the opposite of courage is not cowardice—it's conformity.

When you blindly conform to rules, every time you do, you weaken your ability to be courageous and with it, you're giving your life up to living in a way that *someone else* decided was a good idea.

The type of "silly little rules" I'm talking about plague society. They restrict progress. They stop people from needing to think, from living of their own free will, or using their own minds to come to their own conclusions about what is right and wrong for their own lives. All things that are a prerequisite for a life of growth and prosperity.

To be clear, rules are different from laws.

If rules stop you from thinking, then laws stop you from going to jail. Feel free to break a few stupid HOA rules about painting your house a different colour, just remember to stop short of irritating police officers by driving 60 miles per hour in a 30 mile per hour zone.

"Think for yourself" is a wonderful idea that I champion, but it's difficult to do with so many "invisible" rules around that are reinforced by society.

Whether it is a rule about when you should marry, when you are supposed to have kids, what you can wear at work or school, the importance of a college degree, the words you can use in conversation, the people you should hang out with, the time you can spend on vacation each year, right down to the rules about retirement and spending, someone made all of these rules up long before you arrived on Earth.

You're even making your own rules up about what you think you *should* be getting from life and how others *should* treat you. This being the fastest route to a life of anger and frustration.

But here's the thing: no matter how important they appear, all rules are there to be broken.

In fact, the only rule you should ever follow is this one: **question all the rules.**

That's because they probably don't apply to how you want to live. They're probably not conducive to an Extraordinary life.

Whoever made the rules could never have known what you want from your life and only you ever will. Whether that is your parents, grandparents, former teachers, family members alive today or who have gone before you, elected officials, or colleagues and peers, none of these people have the right to tell you what rules you should and shouldn't be following. Only you should decide that. Anyone who tells you otherwise is more interested in preserving their own view of the world, than they are you discovering it for yourself.

That person's involvement in your life probably needs limiting or at the very least closely inspecting for just how much it's holding you back.

Good Guilt? Or Bad Guilt?

So why do rules work so well to keep people conforming in the first place? And how have we got so many of them in life?

The first is that following rules makes living life much easier. Rules provide a shortcut that the brain can follow, making it less taxing and generally easier to go about making it through life. There's lots of energy expended in thinking, so if there's a rule for something, it's much easier to follow it. It's why so many people love rules and always want more. It means they don't have to think. Literally.

The second reason rules work is because you feel *guilty* about breaking them.

In Chapter One I wrote about the guiding principle that in one way or another, we're all on a quest to *feel better about ourselves*. The problem is feeling guilty is something that gets in the way of that feeling good about yourself. It means people will do anything to avoid guilt, right down to following stupid rules made up by someone whom they've never even met.

Guilt is one of the biggest tricks the media and politicians play to coerce people into following their ways of thinking. You might know in your own mind that the rules you're being asked to follow seem pretty dumb, or simply don't make any sense. But when faced with the choice of feeling guilty about breaking them, or the frustration that comes from following along blindly, most people will accept frustration every time. It's a lot less potent.

Guilt plagues most people all their lives.

No matter what they do, people feel guilty about something. Guilty about being at work, guilty about *not* being at work. Guilty about spending time with one kid, not enough with the other. Guilty about spending money on the family, guilty about not spending money on the family, even guilty about *not feeling guilty*.

Heck, most people feel guilty about being happy. Talk about messed up!

Left to its own devices, guilt does most of the work of keeping you stuck in life. That's why if you're planning on leading an Extraordinary life—or simply getting to the next level in your life—you're going to have to know how to deal with this thing called guilt. Ideally, make it irrelevant in your life. It can be someone else's problem if they want it, but not yours.

It starts by accepting that you can.

So how do you do it? Just how do you rid yourself of the thing that is probably troubling your thoughts and feelings all day, every day?

First up, acknowledge that there's two different types of guilt.

There's *good* guilt and there's *bad* guilt.

Good guilt is when your kid tells you that "they miss you" or "don't want you to go to work." It might not be nice, but really, this is great!

Why? Because if you're going to be missed by someone it means you're *significant* to someone. The feeling you get should serve as a nice reminder of just how important you are to someone. Basically, re-wire what it means.

There'll be a day in a few years where that same person doesn't even notice you're not in the house and you'll wish it were different.

And what is an example of *bad* guilt?

It's any situation where you're *letting yourself* feel bad because of a set of judgemental eyes having been placed upon you. If your kid wanting you to stay at home to watch a movie or play soccer is an example of good guilt, then bad guilt is your mother-in-law suggesting you should stay at home simply because you being at work on the weekend doesn't fit with *her* view of the world and your role in it. It goes without saying that the latter should be eradicated from your life.

Not necessarily your mother-in-law—that is optional and up to you—but definitely the part where you think you have to feel bad because of what she says or suggests.

The trick is to notice when you feel guilty, and then ask yourself which one you're experiencing. Is it good guilt, or is it bad? Use the negative feeling you get from guilt to ask better questions about why you feel that way and make a real time decision about what you need to do because of it. It may be true that this time you *do* need to stay and watch the movie, but I doubt it's true every time.

The next thing to dilute or eradicate guilt is to commit to a way of living that allows people a *bit of rope* in how they behave, as well as what they say or do, so that you can give yourself that same length of rope too.

Let me explain:

Although you won't always want to agree, especially not in the heat of an argument or disagreement, the reality is most people are responding to any given situation with the best way they know how.

It means when other people do something to upset you, they're not necessarily doing it on purpose. It's not an attack on you. It's their best attempt to deal with the situation in the best way they know possible, at that time. If the situation isn't handled well, at best, all it does is expose a part of them that perhaps needs developing. Examples being *restraint*, *detachment*, or better *critical reasoning* skills.

And it's the same for you.

However you reacted and however you behaved, you handled it the best you knew *at that time*. It doesn't mean you are a bad person or that with hindsight you couldn't have or wouldn't have wanted to do better, but however you react, it is usually with what you know and the best you know. Otherwise, you *would* have done it differently.

It also helps to understand that when you fall out with someone or argue over something, all that is happening is one person is violating a *rule* that the other set.

Not a rule like a rule of law, but a self-made, invisible rule, for how they think others *should* behave. And because most of us don't trot out our rules for how we expect to be treated every time we meet someone, it means arguments and disagreements with other people can happen very easily.

They're also usually spontaneous. Which doesn't always bode well for pleasant, well-rounded discussions where both parties get their points across peacefully and calmly, tolerant of the other person's position. As you will probably know only too well, it's quite often the opposite.

And it's this instant, often less than flattering, reaction that most people feel guilty over. As an aside, if you know someone who spends all their life arguing with others, the reason they do so regularly is because they've created lots of rules for how they think they *should* be treated by others.

And on the other side of the coin, the person who *never* seems to be in a disagreement and hardly ever falls out with anyone, that person has very few, if any self-created rules. It's hard to violate a rule that doesn't exist and so this person is rarely ever going to be arguing with others.

As a general rule, it's the people with too many rules, and who always want even more rules, that have the most issues and conflict in life. Not to mention frustration. It's why people in positions of power, on the boards of things like homeowners' associations etc., who love to make up and enforce rules, are often the most miserable, negative, and live mostly in conflict. These people are an unconscious victim of their *own rules about rules* and the punishment—in the form of the constant *conflict* they feel—can't change until they change the way they see life.

Anyway, why is this important to understand and eventually accept?

It's because of this very simple fact, dear reader: if giving other people a *bit of rope* is good enough for them, it's sure good enough for *you*.

Think about it. If all they did was what they knew at the time, all you ever did was the best that you knew at the time as well. If it's fair and reasonable to cut someone else slack on the "rules" that were violated that affected you, why isn't it true for you and any rule breaking that you might want to do or have done? You probably didn't know their rules as much as they didn't know yours.

This is a simple, amicable solution to freeing yourself from guilt that works on both parts. I'm basically saying, "Hey, whatever you did, no worries. I'm OK with it." And, by the same token, "Whatever I did, I'm OK with that as well." It doesn't mean you forget whatever it was the other person did, or that you are immediately best friends again. You just learn to accept it and move forward regardless.

The same is true of yourself. You might never forget that you hurt someone, but you now carry it with you differently. It's to learn from but not to beat yourself with every single day.

If you don't want to do that, my second, more candid piece of advice is this: exercise your right to feel precisely how you want to feel in this life and simply choose to opt out of guilt. Whoever is judging you, screw them all. Flip the middle finger to everyone who ever believed you did something wrong and is holding it against you.

No one has any right to judge you—so don't let them. Their judgement is irrelevant.

People will never know the context of why you did what you "did" and most will never take the time to ask or find out why. Go ahead and tick the box that says you're exempt from guilt just because you can.

And if you ever feel guilty about doing that, ask yourself this: Who would ever know that you don't feel guilty? I won't tell anyone if you don't.

"I'm Not Riding On The Golf Course"

I believe what most entrepreneurs really want from starting their business is more *autonomy* in their life. They won't use that exact word, but that's what they crave: the ability to be independent in their thoughts and actions. Free to *be*, *do* and *think* exactly how they want and not dictated to by elders or society.

@THEPAULGOUGH

A lack of autonomy is the true cause of the frustration that people feel when they describe never feeling like they're in control of their lives, no matter how old they are or how much money they've got. The lack of autonomy comes from a life where rules, well, rule.

These rules are not necessarily written into an official policy or regulation, but they are there, hovering over us all, waiting for the next sucker who comes along to obey without question. It doesn't even have to be as serious as the expectations about your career or your marriage plans—they can be much more subtle. Or much more stupid, if you prefer.

One of my favorite *stupid rules* is the one that says kids should board an aircraft *first*.

I travel a lot. I'm on and off planes with my kids all the time and I can't for the life of me work out why it's in anyone's best interest to get the kids on first. Whoever made that rule obviously doesn't have kids.

How on earth is it a good idea to strap two-year-olds into a seat thirty minutes longer than everyone else? By the time the plane takes off it's no wonder it resembles a maternity ward that has run out of milk. All of the same kids who dutifully boarded the plane first are now screaming to be released from their seat belts.

There are even stupid rules forbidding you from walking or riding your bike on the grass—and worse, people try to enforce them.

True story: I often ride my bike to get to the centre of town where I live in Celebration, Florida. I take a short cut across the golf course each time I do (gasp!). This one time I was stopped by a drab looking official from the golf club who asked me bluntly, "What do you think you're doing?"

In an instant I told *him*, "*Saving fifteen minutes.*"

He furiously told *me*, "I couldn't do that."

I immediately assured him that I *could*, as I do it almost every night.

I told him that if I went the long way round it would take much longer and given that I am often going to meet a friend of mine for a beer, that's not ideal.

Anyway, his communication got a bit better and told me what he really meant was that I couldn't ride on the golf course as "it is not allowed." Someone, somewhere said so.

I reminded him that I wasn't riding "on the golf course" as I was on the concrete path that traversed the golf course reserved for the type of vehicle he was driving in. I pointed out that he was on the same path as I and boldly asked him "what's all the fuss was about?"

He went on to tell me there was a *rule* about not being on the golf course and even pointed to a sign in the distance telling people to keep off it.

We agreed to disagree about me being "on" the golf course, as technically I wasn't, and I told him that although I respected his sign, I thought it a bit over the top. A polite way of saying it's rather pointless. I told him signs like that were open to interpretation and I concluded that in my interpretation I wasn't doing any harm in spite of the sign's presence.

Now the point of the story is not to offend any avid golfers who are reading this book, and probably screaming at me right now for my lack of respect for their game. No, it's a reminder of how even though rules may exist, they don't always make much sense.

I'm also suggesting that you should never be afraid to challenge the rules or the tedious individuals trying to enforce them.

When you look around, these type of signs are everywhere. Signs stopping kids playing soccer in the street or forbidding people walking on grass.

There must be someone, somewhere, with a really big business printing these stupid signs to enforce these stupid rules. Right now, that person is about to hear from another one of those jumped-up employees at one of those pointless homeowners associations.

There he is, waiting patiently for a request for a sign that will keep kids from enjoying life, playing ball games on a road or against a wall, and he's likely making a fortune doing it. Every day, printing more signs, with more people stopped from enjoying life, playing ball games, walking on grass, playing on fields, cycling on country roads and the like. It's madness.

But it keeps on happening.

It's as if they are all thinking the answer to all the problems they have in life is to add more rules to it. They're probably thinking, *I'm miserable and unhappy, it must be because there aren't enough rules in this world. Let's get another one in place.*

Honestly, I'd love to be in that same factory for a day. After receiving a request for another sign forbidding kids playing soccer in the street, I'd send the sign back with the following on it:

"If you're not happy with kids playing soccer here, feel free to go for a *long* walk off a *short* pier. You will probably be happier at the other end."

(A British phrase for reminding someone if they're *that* unhappy with their life there's a way to end it quickly and easily.)

Is It Time to Start Breaking A Few Rules?

@THEPAULGOUGH

I've already started having the conversation with my kids about breaking a few rules. I am not with them 100 percent of the time, so they do from time to time get infected with this highly contagious disease of rule following.

Call me a bad parent if you wish, or anything else for that matter, but I actively go out of my way to tell my kids that they *should* break a lot of rules—and that it is healthy to do so!

One of my favorite moments was the day that my six-year-old son was asked by his basketball coach if following rules was a "good thing."

There were about twenty kids or so in a circle on the floor when the coach asked. In a heartbeat, every single one of the kids raised their hands in agreement. Every one, except for one. That was my boy, Tobias. I looked at him as he looked back at me, and we both had a wry smile on our faces as we both shook our heads to say "No." It was a real proud dad moment.

I'm of the belief that it's simply *not true* that following all rules, without question, is a good thing for anyone. Six-year-olds included. Don't forget that six-year-olds very quickly become twenty-six-year-olds and they bring the habits from childhood into adulthood. Leaving school doesn't come with an automatic wiping of their childhood habits. As I always say, adults are much like kids only with a bit of arthritis in their joints.

Anyway, at the very least, by breaking a few rules occasionally they're developing the muscle of *thinking for themselves*. Which is priceless. Even if they do a few things I'm not overly impressed with at the time, it is more important that they are becoming independent thinkers.

For that reason, I openly encourage them to do a few things their teacher wouldn't approve of or that their grandparents might not think appropriate. It's all under the banner of allowing them a box to play in that is their own. It allows more freedom for them to play and push boundaries to find their own limits, not society's. It is about *containing*, not controlling.

With that said, I wonder if it's high time for you to start breaking a few rules?

You're never too old to start and today is as good a day as any. Especially if your life has somehow flatlined. A plateau in life is the hallmark of too much rule following.

Perhaps you've made great progress in life and business up to this point but now you're somewhat stuck and your life has stalled?

Perhaps you've done as you've been told by people you respect and yet you're still stuck at a place that isn't where you assumed you would be? Perhaps you followed society's rules and achieved society's "dreams" but no matter what you do, you are still not enjoying life and feeling good about yourself? If you *are* at this point in life, maybe it's time to make a decision?

I think there's only two options:

Option 1: Accept and be at peace with continuing down the same path with a life of conformity, saddled with regret, and never knowing what you might have achieved or who you could have become.

Option 2: Get the *brass balls* out and have some fun swinging them around, breaking a few of the rules that are keeping you stuck and in doing so push on to the next level where you make your own rules, have more fun, and make more money.

Well, which will you choose?

If it's the latter, and the *big-old-brass-balls* are coming out, the good news is that you can still respect the rules even if you don't follow them.

Candidly, I respect all the rules—and the people who made them—but I came to my own conclusion that they weren't made with me in mind. That way if my friends or family want to live by the rules, I'm happy for them.

If, year after year, they want to get on that plane first and fight with their kids before take-off, just to conform to the airlines' stupid rules, good for them. Just don't expect me to be at the front of the line with them. I much prefer to be last and hear my name called over the speakers in the departure lounge than have my kids screaming and trying to get out of their seats as we set off on a nine-hour flight across the Atlantic.

If my friends or family want to limit their time on vacation to seven days per year—because that is the accepted rule in their world—then they can go for it. I won't question their view. Just don't expect me to follow suit and don't start to question my way of living when I'm pushing seventy days per year in foreign countries with my kids.

As for pulling them out of school, I'll happily take the fine or the "telling off" from the principle. There's a lot more to be learned on the road than in any classroom and what's funny about that is every teacher knows it's true.

I often wonder what they're *really* thinking as they criticize parents for pulling kids out of school to travel. But now that I've thought about it a little more, I think I have the answer, which is of course, "not much."

After all, they're just following the rules set by someone else.

As for retirement?

Why would I want to retire from doing something I love? Retirement as a goal was an amazing idea when people had the type of physical jobs that meant you couldn't do the work later in life. But in today's society, where most of us sit in offices and behind desks—and now in the comfort of our own homes—how can the rule still be true?

How are we allowed to admire basketball and football coaches working well into their seventies and sometimes eighties, but we're still allowing everyone else to believe they have to stop at sixty-five? I respect retirement. I'll prepare for it just in case I'm physically incapable of working later, but anything I put aside today for the future is nothing more than worst case scenario planning.

I think the best part of rule breaking is that it can be a lot of fun.

In the end, you start to love doing it and you really can get a kick out of rule breaking just by paying attention to the reactions of the people who are offended by you doing so.

Learn to love breaking rules because you know it will send the jumped-up homeowners association manager off like a firework on July 4 when you paint your door pink without asking his permission. This would be a great way to, as we say in Britain, "Put the cat amongst the pigeons." That is to go out of your way to cause a bit of trouble, and often for your own amusement and pleasure.

As an aside, one of the best reasons to get rich is you can do it from time to time without caring too much about the consequences.

Anyway, when he comes along to ask about the paint on your door, simply reply, "What door?". Don't make any mention of the color and don't apologize. Just keep asking, "What door, I don't see a door. It must be my eyes. I'll have to get them checked out. Thanks for bringing this to my attention."

See how long you can keep up the charade before the jumped-up little twit (a British term for "asshole") realizes he's talking to someone who has no interest in playing the stupid games those tyrants want to play.

To finish him off completely, as he walks away, ask him to place the empty pink paint can in your trash at the end of the drive on his way back to his car. That'll really push him into the coronary ward. It'll also be worth any penalty he gives you. Just take it out of your entertainment budget for that month.

I can't stress enough that there are so many ways of living that are out of date that you need to be conscious off.

Most are probably being passed on to you by your parents, who had them passed on to them by their parents, and so on. Fine. I love that. It's admirable. That is what parents naturally do. Following rules is what people like to do to feel safe and that's the natural instinct of any parent—to keep their kids safe.

But when some of the rules we're living by in the twenty-first century were invented by someone living in the 19th century, who knew nothing of the internet, air travel, great healthcare, knowledge-based work over manual labour, communicating with the world via a device in your hand, and even the ability to educate yourself from a free app, how can we possibly still be living by those same rules? It doesn't make sense to me.

I think the real issue for most people is not who is in charge of the country or their lack of money, it is that so many people are literally living in a period of time where abundance and opportunity are everywhere but are being bound by rules that were relevant for a period of time when the only way to be rich was being born into it. Like 16th Century Britain.

Heck, you couldn't even win the lottery back then and you probably couldn't even rob a bank to get rich, as they didn't exist when half of society's rules were made up. You definitely couldn't take out your iPhone, upload some videos to YouTube, and a few weeks later get paid millions by Google for doing so.

I believe the stress that so many people report living with is the resistance that they feel coming from being pulled between the two worlds of opportunity and living by these life-limiting rules. They can see others seizing an opportunity, but they can't get a break. And it's bugging the life out of them. Their only solution is to do more of what didn't work in the first place—follow more rules made to keep the masses average.

The "Rules" of Business

So, what's all this rule breaking got to do with entrepreneurship and running a business? Well, there are silly and outdated rules in business, just like there are in society. Whether it's rules about when you can start the business, how old you must be, or how much experience you need, there are rules waiting for you to follow that someone created years back.

Apparently, there are rules about how business owners must dress, rules about impressing your peers, and behaving "appropriately" and in accordance with how your profession wants you to represent them. There are even rules about the economy, about what people will pay and what they won't pay in "your town."

There are rules about pricing your services, how many hours you must work, and how *few* times you can go on vacation. There are even rules about marketing and sales and what you are allowed to say or do before being deemed "sleazy" by your peers or competitors.

Basically, there are loads of rules that business owners are supposed to abide by but, quite frankly, most of them are ridiculous.

How do I know that?

Simple. Just like most people are not truly happy or fulfilled, most businesses are not successful. The results of conforming don't lie. The facts are that, on average, 50% of businesses go bust within the first five years of opening and 96% of businesses are not there after ten. Only 4% of businesses make it to year ten and only 1% ever make it to $1,000,000 or more. Those are not great results.

That's why I can confidently say that the generally accepted rules of business ownership do not work. The biggest job on your hands is not being seduced into following the rules of the *poor* and that will be hard because almost everyone around you will be sticking to them. The pack is hard to exit even in the business owner community.

But make no mistake, if you're planning on getting to the next level in your business, you are going to have break rules and love doing so. I suggest making rule breaking in your business your new hobby.

Why don't you start by arriving at work in a pair of Hawaiian swim shorts, remove the phone from your office, and hand your office keys back to the staff? Tell them you are doing a little spring cleaning and you decided the door keys were pointless—you don't plan on being there early or late enough to ever need them. Someone else can open and close the office from now on.

Ask your staff to *delete* your phone number. Explain that from now on they have to call your *partner* to get to you in the event of an emergency. That should make them think twice before calling you to ask what to do about the coffee machine that broke while you're on vacation.

Block out all the summer months that your kids are out of school. If anyone asks what your plans are, tell them you haven't decided what you're going to do with those days yet, but that it's going to be something very important. It's either the beach in Spain or a yoga retreat in Hawaii, but you don't know yet. You will decide the *night* before.

And if clients ask why you're wearing Hawaiian swim shorts in freezing-cold January, tell them it's because it's cold outside and wearing summer shorts makes you feel a little warmer.

Honestly, the hardest thing will be to do it all with a straight face.

All of this is fun, my type of fun, partly because most people don't know you're doing it so seriously do they take life (more on this in Chapter 5). But it's important to remember that there's a difference between outdated rules and what I will call "best practices". You should ignore stupid rules, laugh in the face of them almost, but you should never ignore best practices.

It would be, well, stupid to do so!

There are best practices for marketing, sales, finance, leadership, etc., and they absolutely must be sought out, understood, and faithfully applied. Do not try to ignore best practices if you're running a business. They are there to accelerate the process of being successful.

This is why you should always be part of a peer group or mastermind-type program, no matter what type of business you run. There's no faster way to find extraordinary success in business than to be part of a group of ambitious peers who meet regularly and are committed to sharing what is and isn't working in your sector.

Seeking out best practices is the only *real* shortcut to business success and that's never going to change. It's why I feel so sorry for business owners who refuse to get into these types of peer-to-peer communities. They often think it's expensive to be part of one—but it's not nearly as expensive as making mistake after mistake in your business.

Truth is, these type of business owners say they want success, but they're not prepared to put their money where their mouth is. They speak the words of ambition but that is about all. They are not really committed to it with action. What is more, these are often the same business owners who don't like spending money and then moan when their own customers won't spend money with them. How ironic! Karma, perhaps?

Anyway, here's the X (formerly Twitter) style version of this chapter: **To get to the next level in life or business, you *cannot* play by the same rules of the people living at the level below you—no matter how harsh that sounds.**

If you want to live a different life, you've got to play a different game.

In doing so, you absolutely will irritate a few people. But that's OK. Remember that it can be quite fun after a while and besides, the ones who seem to care about it don't matter, and the ones who *do matter*, won't care that you are. (Read that last part again. It could be a good way to weed a few people out of your life who perhaps shouldn't be there.)

In the end, having fun breaking rules becomes part of the reason for doing it. As long as you're not breaking the law, learn to have a lot of fun breaking some pointless rules. If you want some practice, or to put something into action immediately, start by announcing that your in-laws are "exempt" from needing to come to your house for the next Thanksgiving or Christmas Day meal.

Tell your in-laws you've had enough of following stupid rules and you've decided the one that means you must *suffer* annually is the first one you're going to break.

See how well breaking that rule goes down before you move on to something a little more adventurous like raising prices and firing staff who are only there because they've always been there. Good luck.

Major Principle of Chapter 2: Following rules keeps you stuck at average and most weren't designed with the type of extraordinary life you want in mind. The only rule is to question all of the rules.

ACHIEVEMENT
CHAPTER 3

Ambition Creates Conflict

You're reading a book about achievement and what it takes to get to the next level of success in your life. An obvious question is, "Why hasn't it happened already?" Why aren't you where you want to be already and feeling like you want to feel more often? This is unlikely to be the first book you've ever read on success.

In fact, I bet you've read dozens if not hundreds of books before this one, not to mention taken classes or been to seminars on the topic of success.

And yet, despite this commitment, I'm going to hazard a guess that you're still not quite satisfied. Perhaps you're not living at what you might call "prime time," nor do you feel ready for it.

Sure, there's probably *some* progress, but maybe it's flatlined or you feel like you're forever going one step forward only to take two steps back?

You make a bit of progress but then something unexpected always seems to crop up, hit you from behind, and knock you out of your groove sending you right back to square one (where ever that even is!).

Why does this happen?

Why, despite investing a significant amount of time and money into your personal development and business growth, do you still feel like you're not making the progress you expected at this point of your life?

Well, the reason is simple to explain but harder to accept.

And here it is: **most entrepreneurs focus on self-development *without* considering what must come first—self-*acceptance*.**

Self-acceptance is the prequel to personal growth. It's OK to read the books on how to improve yourself or grow your business, but there can never be a real and sustainable difference in the quality of your life without first accepting who you are.

Think about it: how can you possibly "grow" yourself if you haven't accepted yourself?

It's like trying to build a skyscraper on top of a shaky foundation. You might get a few stories high but it's always going to collapse in the end. Sadly, this is what is happening to most people who opt for personal growth *before* personal acceptance.

Personal growth tends to take you toward the things you're comfortable with. If you like sales, you study it. If you like marketing, you learn it. If you like finance or the psychology of human behavior, you devour it. If you have that desire to learn, and you want to grow, you have a tendency to look for the things that you're easily excited by. It means your life is fine as long as you're dealing with something that you're comfortable with.

However, the minute you're taken into an area that isn't your sweet spot—for example, hiring or firing, staff quitting, raising prices, dealing with customer rejection, or even judgement from your family about the hours you put in at work—then you're not as secure in yourself and this lowers how you feel about yourself.

Instead of facing the situation head on, full of certainty and optimism about who you are and the journey you're on, you are stopped in your tracks while you work through how you *feel* about the situation.

And it's here, in situations they're not comfortable with, that people lose progress in life. They're feeling bad about themselves and they're trying to work through *that*. They're not working on something important or meaningful, all of their time and energy is being spent on working out how they feel *about feeling bad.*

When that happens, you're not dealing with the original situation anymore. You're now dealing with *how you feel about how you feel*. It means you're not looking for a solution to the original problem, but the one it created. That is how you feel.

To put it simply, it means most people walk round looking for solutions to *how they feel about things* and not an answer to the problem they had that made them feel that way in the first place.

For example, someone criticizes them at work and instead of asking for ways to get better at work, that same person looks for ways to change how they feel about the comments. Usually with copious amounts of alcohol, narcotics, a credit card, or a rant on Facebook. Perhaps even a face-to-face confrontation to ask them to take the criticism back. All perfectly common in todays day and age.

But it also explains why so few people make real progress in life. Everyone is fixing the wrong problems.

The other thing to be aware of is how people try to solve the new problem they've created. They try to do so by *thinking* it. They're trying to think themselves into feeling better. Which simply isn't possible. No one can ever make himself feel better just by thinking about it.

It's why so many people report feeling lost. They literally go into their own heads and never come out. They go in and get stuck up there, going round and round trying to work out why they feel bad and what to do about it, all the while reinforcing how bad they feel.

As much as people like to try, you can't go into your head to get a logical solution and try to solve an emotional problem. It just doesn't work. You can solve a logical problem at work by thinking it through, but not one about how you feel. You only ever get stuck in a horrible thought loop as you try that creates lots of pent-up energy but no real answer. This is where "over thinking" comes from and it creates pent-up energy known as stress or anxiety.

And, as you know, it's not good for feeling great about life. More often than not the only way to rid yourself of it is to get angry or let it out another way. Tears, for example.

A Feeling of Absolute Certainty

Solid buildings need a solid foundation and you and I are no different. The type of solid foundation that I'm talking about here is a feeling of absolute certainty—safety and security—that comes from accepting a very simple fact:

who you are *already* is good enough to deal with *anything* that is thrown at you as a result of the life you want to live or the decisions you make.

I believe problems and setbacks give you the confidence to know you can deal with other such things that will inevitably come along later in life. By working through the problem, you prove to yourself that although you didn't want the problem, you *can* deal with it.

And when you realize this, and embrace your ability to deal with unwanted situations, you begin to realize just how capable you are of succeeding in this life.

Acknowledging that you are someone who can deal with problems allows you to bounce through life, walking much taller and more confidently knowing you have the greatest skill of all that anyone in life can get; the ability to handle the adversity and setbacks that life inevitably throws at you.

If people just realized this, most would instantly feel better about the future. If people faced up to their problems and looked at them as them as tests they'd passed to get to this point in life, their outlook would be very different. It would be much less fearful and worrisome, that is for sure.

Instead of fretting about another problem that will inevitably come along, they'd feel great about themselves knowing that when it does, it's going to be fine because they'll back themselves to get past it. And why wouldn't they? They've done it before!

And that's the trick to dealing with problems that people are missing. They're not giving themselves enough credit, using and even leveraging their proven resilience, to be able to live a better, more secure life. Instead of always thinking *Why me?* or *Here we go again*, it would be *I'm ready for this, let's go.*

It's another one of those things that confuses people.

Problems are not nice. The only real issue is that people think they shouldn't have any. But as much as they are unwanted, they're a fact of life.

The key is to remember that as each one happens, it's *you* who gets to decide how you want to deal with it and how it's going to affect you.

Contrary to what most people think, I strongly disagree that life and the events of it shape you. Most people want to believe that the events of life are what shapes your life, but I think the opposite. I believe *you* shape your own life with how *you* decide to meet and deal with whatever life throws at you. If you get some bad or unexpected news, that is one thing.

But it's what *you* do next that matters most and not the bad news someone else delivered. It's not the circumstances of the problem, it's how *you* decide to deal with them. Your life isn't created by circumstances it's by your handling of the circumstances.

For example, if you find out that someone has stolen from you at work, one option is you *could* spend your whole life worrying it will happen again and never hiring anyone else, sentencing yourself to a lifetime of being tied to your office. Option two is you choose to accept that *you* made a bad decision to give someone too much control of your money, unsupervised, and knowing that you played a part in it, act differently in future so it doesn't happen again.

Highlight this next sentence: **thinking that life shapes you is a *passive* way of living**. A way that means you will never feel in control.

Shaping your own life by deciding you will handle what it throws at you is an *active* way of living. A way that even puts you in control of events you might deem *out of your control*—the type that really dictate to the circumstances of your life—and allows you to learn from everything. It's a "win or learn" type of mentality that should be etched into your thinking about life.

If the quality of your life is dictated by your beliefs, then surely the *ultimate belief* to carry with you is the one that says you're able to control how you react to anything that happens to you?

It's to see an event as happening *for* you and not *to* you.

Whatever it is, it's to see it as something you *get* to do, not something you've *got* to do. It's not easy, but it's 100% possible. And you must at least try.

If you follow how the masses think and you believe that life events shape you, you'll always be at the mercy of those events. Life will carve out its own picture of you and in the end you will become someone you hardly recognize. You'll look in the mirror and see a shadow of the person you *intended* to become, never able to work out at what point you lost or gave up on the life you *intended* to live.

Eventually, you'll start to believe that whatever happens in life is because fate picked on you—as if you're a victim. Which, if I may say so, is how a lot of people live their lives. With a victim mentality.

It's always about them and how they feel about things, how whatever it is has affected their life, and it's always in a way that no one else can ever understand. All fine and valid. But what they don't realize is that this is precisely why they *suffer* so much.

When you make it about you, and how you feel about it, it's suffering. However, when you separate the problem from how you feel about it, sure, it's still going to be painful, but that's not nearly as difficult to deal with as suffering.

Yes, I'm sure there's an element of fate in all our lives, but not so much that you should give your entire life over to it as though someone has already dictated your path.

I believe you absolutely can live life on *purpose* and you do that by meeting any situation you are in with the attitude that, whatever it is, you will commit to making the best of it. It's all you've got. It's all you need. The commitment to decide whatever it is, even if Lady Luck wasn't shining the day you started your business and COVID shut everything down the next day, you will make the best of it.

I believe that one of your most important jobs is to make your reality better than any twist of fate. No matter what anyone tells you, you absolutely can change your own *view* of reality and then work to make it *become* a reality. That's how you make progress in your life.

That's also what the best entrepreneurs really do.

They create a reality in their minds *first* and then work to make it an actual reality soon after. When people ask if they're surprised they created it, whatever it was, they usually aren't. They were able to see it in their heads long before and it felt so real that it almost was. They did the work and eventually reality caught up. It was then others got to see what they could see all along—the entrepreneur's dream.

If you ask me, to think any other way than you are able to live it on purpose, is pointless. Maybe that is the real purpose of your life? To live it literally, on purpose.

@THEPAULGOUGH

The Big Problem For Ambitious Entrepreneurs

I believe the best way to make it through this life is by backing and believing in *yourself*. If you have that, you have a real chance of success. You have a shot at a quality of life that is rich both inside and out.

But that isn't what we're allowed to believe. That's not what society tells us about how it works. Instead, we're mostly taught that we must depend upon others for everything we want—including happiness, safety, approval and recognition. We're made to believe that we're never good enough to do or achieve anything alone. And that's just by the government.

It's not possible to sort your own life out—you need the government to do it for you. Or at least that's what they want you to believe (and sadly, many do!).

We're told that our only chance of being happy is if you marry the *perfect* partner and have *perfect* kids like you see in Hollywood movies.

We're told that you must go to an expensive college and get a fancy degree or you're deemed a "dropout." There's no other way to learn and apparently "*it matters*" what college you go to. At least that's what my *nine-year-old* was told by his friend at school.

You should have seen the pressure release from his little face when I told him, "No son, it really *doesn't*!"

And if you're still single at twenty-five, wow, there's *surely* something wrong with you. There *must* be something wrong with you if you're still footloose, carefree, and single in your twenties. You simply can't be happy on your own. That's not how it works. You must get a partner to cozy up with every night and never be apart from and if you've not done it by twenty-five, you'll be left on the shelf.

Of course, there really isn't anything wrong and you won't be left on the shelf. It's just society *expects* you to get married early and is confused if you don't. This is mostly because everyone else get married early so there's an expectation to follow suit and, oh yes, some old romantic in the government decided it was better for your kids if you do.

Apparently, your kids will be happier and are guaranteed to be raised in a loving home because of it. They'll even give you a tax break for doing so.

Who said romance was dead?

All of this is complete nonsense, not to mention mostly unattainable. Whether it's marrying to try to guarantee happiness, going to college to get a better job, or needing other people's approval of how kids are raised, this is what droves of people are buying into as their blueprint for happiness.

They're looking for someone to validate how they live and that's the reason it doesn't work.

It's why so many are unhappy despite being married, or have big incomes after college but are still miserable as they try to pay off student loan debt. It's madness, but at the same time it's not. It's actually really easy to explain: **we live in a world where most people are *emotionally dependent* upon what others think about them in order to feel good about themselves.**

That's why millions of people get married when they have *doubts*.

It's why they go to college even though they don't want to.

They're doing it because they need validation and approval from someone other than themselves. Usually their parents. It's gotten so bad that it seems to me that most people have decided that the purpose of their lives is to be approved of by others. It's a sad but very real and common scenario.

And therein lies the big problem for any ambitious entrepreneur like you.

If you're living with an *unconscious* need for validation and approval from others around you, to feel good about yourself and what you're doing, then this game of business you're playing will tear you to pieces from the inside out.

Many entrepreneurs like to think of themselves as "different"—and in many ways they are. The fact that they want to work for themselves and take all the risks associated with that is the biggest sign they're a bit, well, strange. Just 10% of the world want to do it. The rest prefer the safety of a steady job.

Despite being "different" in that respect, you're not different in that you're automatically immune from the friction that inevitably comes from doing what is required to run your own business.

What do I mean by this?

Well, you're committed to a life of growth. Your ambition is relentless, and yet most of the people around you are content with a life of safety and comfort, thinking and doing mostly the same things they did the day before. Living for forty years on paper, but in reality, just one year, forty times over.

The bit in between how *you* want to live and how *they think* you should live is this friction. And you will feel any time they question why you're going to work on a weekend or getting on a plane and spending money on *another* business seminar. They'll never get what drives you on or how you can happily do what you do. They can never quite grasp why you love going to work when they want to rush home from it and what is more, it'll likely irritate the life out of you that they don't.

But, and however tempting it is, you cannot behave like everyone else.

Remember that someone who wants to make a six-figure salary has a very different set of behaviors and thoughts than someone striving to makes seven figures. Someone who wants ten weeks' vacation per year thinks radically different than someone who *accepts* two weeks.

The problem is that the people around you don't understand this. They're part of a larger network of friends and colleagues who are telling each other that life is about following rules, working hard, and waiting in line for someone to tell them it's their turn for a promotion at work or when they can go on vacation.

They erroneously believe they can get to the next level by doing what they've always been doing, but just working a bit harder at it. It's the popular belief that most people buy into.

But why wouldn't they believe such a thing? After all, we've all been raised by our parents to "work hard and do a good job."

I know I was.

Don't get me wrong, hard work is important. And following the rules is fine, at least for a few years. But ask anyone who is already where you want to be—at the next level—and I bet they won't tell you they got there by *just* working a bit harder or following rules.

It's more likely they'll tell you it was because they worked hard at first, then they behaved and thought *radically* differently than everyone else around them. They put a great work ethic behind that radical thinking and rule breaking, but it wasn't simply a case of working more hours or any harder.

There is much more to success than that and one of those things is the ability to deal with *conflict*. And lots of it. It's why the journey you're really on is to find a way to balance how you feel about yourself, and what others think of you, with your own ambition. It's going to come up at many points in this book.

When most people around you are happy with average lives, average incomes, and average lifestyles, and you're loaded with ambition, there's going to be some level of conflict that you must know how to deal with.

That's why I say that *ambition creates conflict.*

Specifically with friends, family, and the world around you in general.

This is why self-acceptance is a must. The friction will heat you up and melt you down if you don't have the ability to believe in yourself and how you're living. Getting that belief is also going to be your *ultimate advantage.*

And here's why: the safety and security you create for yourself is what really makes the difference in life. It's not a college degree—everyone has one of them and most aren't worth the paper they're written on. It's not the money you will make, either. That comes *after* you create the security in yourself. People are attracted to your security and they want to pay you for it.

The trick is to realize that being secure in yourself is something you must activate first—before you're ready—and doing so allows you to deal with conflict and advance in uncomfortable situations, regardless.

You do not activate self-belief when you get rich. You activate it *to* get rich. You don't *become* courageous when you've tackled a risky situation. You've got to *behave* courageously *first* and *then* you get to call yourself a courageous person. Everything you want is on the other side of the action that it requires.

Anyway, I put it to you that how you react and deal with this inner conflict will determine how far you go in business, and it'll also have a big say in how you enjoy your life. If you're using energy on fighting inner conflict then it's *not* being used for ideas, creativity and progress. All of which are vital tools for an entrepreneur to have at their disposal.

This brings us nicely to the next, very important point.

When Does The Day Arrive?

So, when does the big day arrive? When will you *finally* feel secure in yourself on a consistent, moment-to-moment basis, unresponsive to the trivial opinions and different beliefs of others around you? When does that day arrive?

Well, it's assumed that being self-assured—having that feeling of certainty about who you are and what you stand for—happens with adulthood and the passing of time or life experience. The theory is some version of, "If I just stay alive long enough, *eventually* I'll get to be confident in who I am just like all the older people around me seem to be."

If only it were that simple.

What happens is as a kid you look at adults and *assume* they have it all figured out. Because they're bigger than you and dealing with adult things, you assume they have this security that you, as a child, don't have yet.

You think it will come with age or perhaps when you get physically bigger. But it never does, does it? If anything, because you *imitated* what they did and how they lived, you end up with what they have. A disease called insecurity.

Even as an adult, you look across the room and *assume* all the other adults have it figured out *except* you. You tell yourself that one day, someday, if you wait your turn long enough (or when you win that lottery), the insecurity will go away and the belief you need to live your own life will finally arrive.

This whole thing goes on and on and is one of life's biggest tricks that the greatest of all magicians would be proud to have invented: the one that has everyone on earth thinking everyone else is secure *except* them. Talk about a self-fulfilling prophecy.

The reality is that just because you made it to adulthood, you don't *automatically* possess the courage and security you crave to do adult things.

Unless you've had a few too many alcoholic drinks or you've taken a substance that your grandmother wouldn't approve of, there *isn't ever* going to be a single day in your life where you just wake up and miraculously feel amazing about yourself—like it's your turn and you've waited long enough. That's not how it works.

The truth is most people live their whole their lives absent of a feeling of internal safety and security. They don't live happily ever after, they mostly live perpetually *insecure*.

Insecurities can show up in your life without any warning.

One day you're feeling good about yourself, but then in comes *that* email with the news about another employee quitting. Now you're back to feeling bad about yourself for weeks on end. "Why are they leaving *me*?" "What did *I* do wrong?" "Am *I* a bad leader?"

These are just some of the questions you've got, and it wouldn't be so bad if you were asking the questions with a view to learning something about yourself. But you're not! You're just reinforcing how bad you feel about yourself in a "poor me" kind of way that gets you nowhere and stifles your progress.

This also reveals one startling fact about you: you take things far too personally.

Whatever happens, you make it about you. You start to inflict that self-imposed suffering and misery I mentioned in Chapter 1.

Your employee is leaving isn't the issue, how you feel about it is. That bad review on Google isn't the issue, how you feel about what you perceive as a personal attack is. That your parents don't appear to give a toss about what you get up to in your life isn't the issue, that you think they *should* is.

Instead of spending time thinking about how to respond to the situation and move forward positively, your thinking turns to how you *feel* about the situation, and, in most cases, it confirms your own *low* expectations for yourself.

You were never certain about your leadership skills, so the minute the resignation comes in or the staff criticize you, it confirms that you were right—you *are* a bad leader.

You were never sure you were a great parent, so the minute your kid disrespects you, it confirms your worst fears—you *are* bad parent. On and on it goes. Whatever it is, the roads always lead back to how you feel about what you think it says about you. That's the bit you need to become aware of and stop. You need to change what you think it all means. Your kid not picking the clothes means he's a kid, who, like all kids, doesn't want to do anything that his parents want him to. That's it!

Anyway, one last thing on this: if you want a litmus test for just how much self-belief you have, simply look at the prices you charge right now.

Entrepreneurs usually set their prices in line with the view they have of themselves. If they feel strong and confident in themselves, their prices are high. If they suffer from low self-esteem, then their prices will be equally as low. And where are most people's prices?

Exactly where most people's self-esteem is: average-low.

If that's you, I propose a change. Let's start with a fair and reasonable increase in your own self-belief, of say 50%. Then let's ask your client's to pay for that with an adjustment in your prices accordingly and immediately.

If clients ask why the hefty price rise, tell them all it's because you've *finally* realized how much you believe in yourself and today's the day you decided to charge appropriately for it.

Ex-Employees Who Have a Vendetta (And A WhatsApp Group!)

Before we finish this chapter, let me make it very clear that I'm not saying personal development isn't important. Personal development is a *vital* part of your progress. It involves getting better at things like marketing, hiring, time management, communication, sales and influence, understanding finance, strategic thinking, creating business plans, etc.

But if you go straight for personal development, you miss the rung on the ladder that gives you the stability to deal with challenges and conflict.

Put another way, and in case I haven't explained the point well enough yet, the quality of your life will stand and fall not by how much money you make, but by how well you can deal with challenges and limit conflict.

@THEPAULGOUGH

It will ultimately be determined by what you focus on and if you're not careful, what you will focus on most is how you *feel* about the challenge or the conflict and not on making the necessary adjustments to get beyond it. There's no point swimming in that pool of cash I mentioned in Chapter 1 if you're always arguing with someone on the phone while you're in it.

Remember that no matter what you do, someone is going to have an opinion on it. And it won't always be favorable. The question is, how will you deal with that?

How will you deal with it when your ex-employees set up a WhatsApp group to criticize your every move? Come to think of it, how will you deal with it when there are *two* WhatsApp groups because you've fired that many people?

And in case you're wondering, *yes* that has happened to me and when it did, I let it be known that I was *flattered* by it. It was such a buzz to have so many groups named "arsehole ex-boss" in my honor.

If any of them get wind of it being mentioned in this book—which they will, as there's at least two of them who can read, and there's also that one who likes to follow my work and *blatantly* copies it—I have no doubt the chatter in these groups will be fired up again.

My ears will be burning again soon enough, I am sure.

Anyway, that's enough of me "poking the bear" and getting myself into *more* trouble, back to *you* and the important stuff.

How will you deal with bad reviews from clients because they didn't like the latest price increase? They want to pay as little as possible and you just want to make enough to pay the bills. There's conflict in between you two opposing views.

@THEPAULGOUGH

How will you deal with having to fire someone who last month you thought was the saviour of your business because they backed you into a corner and asked for a crazy pay rise that was unsustainable? How will you react when your best employee leaves you and takes your best clients with her?

All these things will test you and there are many more tests coming that you're not expecting. If you're living in fear of what other people think, it's impossible to make the big decisions that you know you need to make.

The books and the coach tell you what to do—they give you the strategy—but for some reason you can't execute or do as you were told. You have all the pieces to the jigsaw puzzle but no clue as to why they aren't fitting together. The creativity is there but the security is not. And that is what people want to be part of. Your creativity *and* your security.

Struggle to keep employees? It's not always because they got offered better pay. They leave because your insecurities expose their own insecurities. They didn't just come to work for a pay cheque, they came to feel safe and secure and they hoped to get that from you. If they don't, they're off to find someone who will give it to them.

This is why life is not *just* about getting a great college education.

It's also why so many people come out of college and still struggle at life. They have the talent (creativity), but they lack the safety and security pieces. They're educated, but they lack a solid foundation and as such live life with that same paralyzing insecurity I spoke about in Chapter 1 that always gets in the way of their progress.

Here's the X (formerly Twitter) style summary: **self-acceptance is the key to growth.**

The best bit is that you don't need anyone else to believe in you except the person looking back at you in the bathroom mirror.

Anyone who tells you otherwise is either trying to keep you trapped, doesn't want you to be independent and free, or is stuck at a level of thinking that is way below the dreams you have for the type of life you want to live. Be careful about listening to such people.

To get to this type of life, all you have to do is accept that it's OK to believe in yourself, that who you are right now is all you need to be right now and it will help to remember this most important of facts whenever you're facing criticism head on:

Most of the people judging you are unable to meet their own expectations of themselves. Why should they ever be allowed to pass judgment on you?

What you get up to or what you choose to do with your life is none of their business and what they think of you for doing so is *none of yours*.

Basically, stay in your own lane and if anyone swerves into it, escort them out ASAP. If they don't leave politely resort to force. Never forget that you never ever need anyone to believe in you but you. Why don't you start today and see how it goes?

If you don't like it, you can always go back to being insecure and miserable. What have you to lose?

Major Principle of Chapter 3: You can't grow yourself until you accept yourself. And only you can do that.

ACHIEVEMENT
CHAPTER 4

What Drives You On Can Also Drive You Mad

If you ask *non*-entrepreneurs what motivates entrepreneurs, most will probably tell you "money." They'd tell you we're all driven to build big businesses, make loads of money, and use it to massage our egos by buying expensive houses and cars.

If only that were true.

If it were, most of us would be significantly happier and more content than we are now. It is not that uncommon for entrepreneurs to have a decent amount of money and yet not all are as happy as they would like.

I started this conversation in Chapter 1 by suggesting that the subject of money and the pursuit of it is easily *misunderstood*. It can sometimes be demonized or weaponized and used against certain people who have a lot of it. As you'll read in a moment, it can even be used to label nice people as "nasty."

In this chapter, I'm going to go a little deeper and find out where this confusion about money and its pursuit really comes from. I'm going to start by suggesting there's an *ignorance* to how people think about money and the role it plays in driving people to do what they do.

The typical person on the street never has enough spare cash and is quick to assume that anyone who does (have some) *must* be motivated by it. There *can't* be any other explanation for how or why someone has built up their wealth than they are "driven by money."

An easy way if ever there was one to justify why there's an absence in their own pocket.

Now their judgment may or may not be correct. But in making such a sweeping assumption, they are neglecting to consider a couple of reasonably plausible scenarios. One is the possibility that the person with the excess cash has a high emotional need to *feel successful*. And in making a commitment to be successful at something such as entrepreneurship has perhaps generated a lot of cash as a *happy by-product*.

The second scenario that people fail to consider is the possibility that the excess cash exists simply because that same person also loves to grow both personally and professionally, and in doing so, moves beyond the *limitations of thinking* that keep most people struggling for cash their whole lives.

The thing that most of the people in the world don't get is that when you have that high need to feel successful, and you commit to personal growth, and then apply both of those attributes to running a business, what comes next is inevitable. That being a lot of the green stuff! Money is a happy by-product of those things being faithfully applied and right now money is how the world has agreed to compensate you for it. To put it simply, money is not the driver, it is often the *result* of the drive.

However, in most people's eyes, that's not how they see it. They think it's all to do with "greed" or an inherent motivation for making money that is found naturally in every rich person's DNA. As if it was formed in the womb before birth.

Personally, I find it a little bit disrespectful when people say such things.

I've had many conversations with different people on this exact subject and I find the ignorance to be stunning. It's as if they're saying, "It's OK for you Paul, you must be motivated by it, but I'm not. It must be in your DNA, but it's not in mine. Poor me. Lucky you. You got golden genes, but my genes have holes in them."

It's obvious that the pursuit of success has a stigma attached to it that is hard for entrepreneurs to shake. Put all your time into being a doctor or lawyer—it's admirable. The family adore you. Put the same time and effort into starting a business—it's because you are rebelling against your up bringing, have aspirations to be a *fat cat* boss addicted to power and money, or a sign that you don't know what you want to do with your life. It's rarely ever positive.

Left unchecked, this stigma can create self-doubt that causes you to question who you are and what you stand for, what your value is and your worth, and none of that isn't great for your self-esteem.

If your parents are questioning why you won't get a "real job" or insinuating that what you do is "all about money," at the very least it can cause you to question your own integrity and credibility. That is no way to live your life. You're not free if you're living like that and you're definitely not going to *enjoy life and feel good about it.*

Let me start by saying that I agree that's there's *some* truth to the idea that entrepreneurs are motivated by money.

But who isn't?

Aren't we're all, in some way or another, motivated to get some of it? There's a reason the poor play the lottery. They want to get in on some of the action.

And why wouldn't they? It can be quite fun being rich.

Fun it may be, but the pursuit of cash is also borne out of a deep-rooted need to survive. And in the most basic of cases, simply stay alive.

Regardless of whether we work for someone, or run a business, we all need a bit of money to be OK in this life. You need money to eat and stay warm and unless you plan on robbing grocery stores for a living and risking going to jail, you're not going to be able to do either. And if you can't eat or stay warm, eventually you're going to end up dead. Which is not good.

So it means we are *all* pretty much in the same boat when it comes to needing a bit of money if for no other reason than to avoid dying from starvation or freezing to death.

The problem with the subject of money is there aren't many people around who really "get it." That is, really understand how it all works.

"Rich People Are All *Nasty!*"

It doesn't help that most of the rich are vilified for being so, which means the type of people society *could* be learning at least *something* from (especially on the subject of how to escape poverty and debt), are instead being ignored and overlooked.

Here's a true story: my nine-year-old son Harry once let slip to me that his friend at school thought all rich people were "nasty." He literally used the word "nasty." He went on to tell me that the kid in school has changed his mind since he met us.

How nice of him.

But also, how naïve of him.

Little does he know that we're good actors in my house and that we all change back to *loathsome, revolting, repulsive* creatures, all counting the money on the bed, the minute he leaves.

Only joking.

(Well, not about the *counting the money on the bed* bit. That I'm never giving up!)

Anyway, I wonder where this nine-year-old kid is getting his view of rich people from in the first place?

And I wonder just how many he's actually met?

I also wonder what amount of money this family decided determines when you can be considered rich (and therefore nasty!) in the first place?

I'd wager that this kid's view is coming straight from his parents.

Fine. But does it *really* help him? Maybe they think it does, but I don't think so.

With a view like this, it means even if there's a good example or lesson to be learned from any rich or successful person this kid meets, it is likely to be missed in favor of thinking that person is somehow inherently bad.

And by the way, why do parents tell their kids that the rich are "nasty" in the first place?

They are preparing the kid for the inevitability of being poor. Like them. It's so the kid can avoid feeling disappointed later in life when inevitably they accept they are not rich themselves.

"That's OK son, we might not be rich, but at least we're not nasty like that lot!"

What it also reveals is how little faith in the kid the parent really has.

Or, how little faith they have in *themselves,* more to the point.

It reveals what the *parent* lacks. That being the belief that the kid *could* live a life that's even a little different or at the level above the one the parent has. Remember in Chapter 1 when I spoke about having curiosity that others in the family don't have? This is exactly what I mean. All someone who is rich ever did was decide to explore what the next level looks like. Their curiosity got the better of them.

In this case, the parent is creating an emotional cushion to ease future disappointment, having already concluded at the age of nine that the kid will never be rich.

How sad. And yet, it's happening all the world over.

Personally, I would choose a conversation with my kid about being rich that went something like this: "If you're planning on being rich, son, first up, good for you. Go for it! You can have a lot of fun with a good bit of cash. The fastest way to be rich is to study the rich and learn from them. Second, just make sure you're rich *inside* as well. Make sure you're a good, decent, and fair human being who treats all people with respect. Because having a

Lamborghini to drive might be nice, but it won't make up for you being an *obnoxious asshole."*

Now I suspect this type of conversation about the rich being "nasty" isn't just happening in my son's friend's house. It's probably widespread, in one version another. So, we can in all probability conclude that there's not that much education on the subject of money coming from parents.

And it's not like we're getting any decent lessons at school either. When the curriculum is created with *average* and *conformity* in mind, there's not a chance of a lesson on *how to think and grow rich* taught by people who actually did it, is there?

Another issue is everyone has their own view of what they deem to be "enough" before you're deemed greedy.

I get it. But the problem is someone's opinion of how much is enough before you're considered greedy, or whatever, is usually based on what *that* person thinks *they'll* need to be happy in *their* life to live the life *they* want.

It's inherently biased and it wouldn't be so bad if they kept it at that, but it's when they assume everyone else should stop at the same level that it becomes a problem. What happens next is really a *conflicting view of ambition*, not money.

What's also interesting, perhaps more revealing than anything else, is that the people who *have* made a lot of money generally seem to want others to do the same. There's no poverty in their minds. Sure, they may not want to give it all away, but they mostly do want others to experience the same and are often more than willing to share how. Often all you have to do is ask.

It is the same with success in business. The ones who are successful seem more eager to want to help others. Interesting, isn't it?

And while we're on the subject of interesting things about money and motivation, here's another: even the people who openly tell you they are only doing it for more money are probably *not* motivated by it.

And this should help you understand why. It's because money, cars, houses, and business success are all about moving *toward pleasure*.

The pursuit of those types of things is about making yourself feel good. And yet, what motivates most entrepreneurs is the complete opposite. We do what we do to *move away from pain*. This is one of the most important things to remember in business and life: that people are more likely to be motivated to do something to avoid or rid themselves of pain than they are to do something that moves them toward pleasure.

Offer your kid five dollars to clean his room and he *might* do it. Tell him you're taking Wi-Fi away for a week and watch how quickly he'll run up the stairs.

Every great marketer knows that if you want a better response from an ad, you must always talk about how your product or service can take the client *out of pain* first.

For example, someone with low back pain is ten times more likely respond to an ad about *avoiding* a life spent in a wheelchair than she is one for the promise of *getting* a good night's sleep.

The same is true with business owners. When the *proverbial* hits the fan they'll suddenly start to make a change to their business for fear of losing it. However, when things are going "OK," it's much harder to get to that seminar to learn what is needed to get to the next level of prosperity.

This is another thing that separates business owners who struggle from those winning. The latter can motivate themselves to keep going regardless of the circumstance and in doing so limit the chance of their ever being a bad time.

With that said, this is where this chapter is about to get very interesting for you. Even if you think you know why you're motivated, what's driving you on, or why you started your business in the first place, I bet there's more going on than you think (there has been with every single business owner I've ever met).

What we're going to try and figure out next is if the drive you've got is a healthy one, or if it's one that is not only going to drive you on, but also *drive you mad*.

Finding Your Why

Discovering what is motivating or driving you is one of the most important things you can ever do in business. Especially if you like the idea of running that business without feeling like you're being *run into the ground*, and no matter how much money you make.

This exercise is popular and is commonly called "finding your why."

There are lots of books written on it and many people recommend you get clear on it before you start your business. The idea is that once you find it you will be more motivated by it and it'll get you back on track whenever you lose your focus.

Your why is designed to get you through the tough times and keep you committed to the task of growing the business through its inevitable ups and downs. It's a popular opinion and I believe that there is a good bit of sense in finding it.

The problem is that the traditional view of "finding your why" only just scratches the surface of what is really needed. It isn't only about finding the motivation to *keep* going. That is one thing.

However, if you want to be *happy*, to feel safe and secure, perhaps even *content* with the progress you're making from your business and in life, then it's also about finding out why you *really started* the business in the first place and ask if it's still driving you now.

I put it to you that *doing that* will be what determines the real quality and enjoyment you experience in your life. It means if you are going to do this "find your why" thing correctly, you've got to find not just one, but *both* of your whys. Here they are:

Easy Why: the one you *think* is motivating you (this is easy and popular, and you'll come up with it in minutes)

Big Why: The one that is *really* motivating you (this one is big and makes you uneasy just thinking of it)

Let me explain them both to you now:

First up, the one you *think* is motivating you is usually something like your kids and the dream of creating a better business for your family. It's nearly always about the future. It's about moving you toward pleasure inspired by the fantasy of a life that is better and more fulfilling for your family than the one you've got now. It's noble and it's fulfilling and makes you feel good about the pursuit of success.

I agree that the obstacles you hit in business (or life) are easier to overcome if you have a vision of you and your kids enjoying a better quality of life. It also allows you to *justify* why you do what you do (instead of getting a "real" job), *defend* why your family is currently living without a good income (as you re-invest in the business), or *rationalize* why you're always at work (instead of home for dinner and story time with the kids).

This "why" has you and everyone around you believing that you're at work on the weekend because you are doing it "for the kids." It's a lovely thought that everyone buys into. It's the type of thing that even makes it hard for your mother-in-law to question what you're doing. After all, it's for the kids! Surely the *old bat* isn't going to deprive your kids of a better future?

She might think you're wrong for working crazy hours, but she's not going to say it out loud and in public if it's "for the kids."

I Am Not Doing It for My Kids (Gasp!)

Personally, I've never needed to rely upon my kids and their future as a reason to go to work. Not because I don't have kids. I've got four of them. And of course, I want them to have a great future. But the reality is if I raise them right and do what I consider my *real* job of being a great father to them, then they'll take care of their own futures, with or without me.

It's why I'm happy to tell you, knowing they could one day read this book, that I am 100 percent doing this business thing for *me*. And I say that guilt free!

I go to work on weekends or stay back late because I *love* the work I do. It's not just to make more money, it's because I love what I do. I get a thrill out of it that's hard to ignore.

I'll say it again: I absolutely *love* running my businesses and here's the news flash that is hard for some people to understand: *that's why I do it!* It's as simple as that. Some people watch football because they love it. I go to work because I love it. Inquest over.

That's also probably also why I am good at it. *Because* I love it, I put all my attention and effort into it. There's no conflict about why I am doing it, so I just go all in on it.

My "easy why" is as simple as the fact that *I love it.*

I have a high emotional need for success, and I scratch that itch through my businesses. I used to love playing teams sports—soccer mainly—and badly wanted to win. I transferred the same need to win over to business ownership and instead of a few medals at the end of the season I ended up with a few million dollars in the bank.

Simple, really. No regrets, either.

Sure, my family gets to enjoy the benefits of my business being successful. And so does Disney. With four kids and living in Orlando, I seem to *spend* most of the success there these days.

I also go to work every day with a smile on my face. And I do so to set an example *to them* and *for them* of how to live their own life and do something that they love, in spite of what others around them might think or say. In *that* way it *is* for them—of course it is—but I make no mistake in saying it is 100 percent about *me*.

That is how the idea behind self-first works. You put yourself first but in doing so you know that the people close to you will really get to benefit from you doing so.

Some might think I am selfish, or weird, or whatever for saying that I do it because I love it, so rare it is to hear anyone talk to so assertively about their work, but better that than me be a liar or someone who lacks the courage to admit the truth. I couldn't stomach being another one of those so called "influencers" telling you do it for your kids, or whatever, when you and I both know it's because we love it.

Here's a radial proposal: If you love your work, stop the charade, and just come out and say so! Stop pussyfooting around and instead of denying it tell people that you *love it* and you consider yourself lucky that you do.

Next question!

And about your kids...

If you're looking to do something "for your kids," why not show them how to live a life where *they too* can do what they love instead of having to justify their choices to others?

That would be a pretty cool gift to give them, don't you think?

That's definitely the way I want my own kids to live. Not waiting for my handouts or to be told by me what to do or not to do. Far from it. I want them to live their own lives and put themselves first and in doing so put themselves in a wonderful position to really help a lot of others for doing so. I want them to be autonomous, free-thinking individuals, as well.

In that respect, this business you're building is still for them, even if it's for you.

They just won't realize it for a few years, and maybe not at all, but when they're living their own lives, inspired by you having the courage to live *your own* life, you'll be the one who gets to sit back and say, "That's really *why* I did it."

And guess what?

That'll probably be your biggest-ever achievement. There'll be a lot of cash in the bank from your business success but that will pale into insignificance when it comes to getting to watch your kids really live their best lives.

Finding The *Big* Why

Now even if you don't agree with *mine*, that I do it because I love it, I am sure you have found your "easy why" by now.

However, the one that most people don't ever know or ever even think about is the second type of why that I like to call *"The Big Why."*

This is the one that fascinates me the most. This is the real and most important "why" in your life and is the one that is probably lurking somewhere in the past, controlling how you feel today, dictating your future. Finding it has been one of, it not *the*, biggest game changers in my own life. If your easy why is about the future, this big one is about the *past*.

It's the why that is causing the incessant need for the business to be successful, at all costs. It's the why that has you always wanting more or something else – even when you're doing well in business and your kids' lives are already better because of it, somehow you're still not satisfied. It's the why that creates the type of life where you're *never happy*—even when all targets have been hit and you've got what you said you wanted from it.

It's the one that creates a *restless* kind of life where you're never content.

It's the one that is not just driving you on—*it's also driving you mad.*

Let me give you the revelation early: what most business owners don't know is that they're often more motivated to rid themselves of pain than they are to get something good. Like I mentioned earlier, it's how most of us are motivated.

What we're talking about here is doing what you do, working silly hours and always wanting more, because you need to rid yourself of a "pain" you've likely lived with since you were a kid. You might not think of it as "pain" in the physical sense, but it's there, scratching at you every day, and in many cases it's worse than physical pain.

People think that the pain from a broken leg is bad. And it is. But it's nothing compared to the pain people live with that comes from *self-doubt, low self-esteem,* and never feeling like anything you do is *good enough.*

Most of us—entrepreneur or not—have this type of thing going on at some level and we all deal with it differently.

Many people turn to things like alcohol, drugs, or adultery or they get into massive debt buying things they can't afford to try and change how they feel about themselves. The instant gratification replaces the low mood associated with that "poor me" feeling we spoke about in the last chapter. But, of course, it never lasts. Hence, they must keep doing it and, in the end, find themselves in a lot of trouble. Massive credit card debt is an example.

The other option is somewhat more positive. It is changing how you feel by trying to *achieve something* or becoming s*omeone.* Starting and running a successful business ticks both boxes. It's assumed the low self-esteem and constant self-doubt will disappear when you can prove to other people that you're good at something distinguished—like owning your own business.

Right or wrong, **most of us entrepreneurs live with the idea that we're not good enough** – no matter how much success we come across.

And in many cases, this is the *real* driver behind the decision to start the business in the first place. This is the real *why* that must be acknowledged if you are to have any chance of a great business—making lots of money—and simultaneously have a *great life* that involves being genuinely happy and content.

This is the bit to understand: having this as your driving force or even your why is fine. At first, that is. But if it remains the same driver years after the money is made and success is achieved, then you're *never* going to enjoy life and feel good about yourself as you live it. If left unchecked, this driver can quite literally run your life, and *ruin it* for that matter, without you even knowing.

It's why I had to bring this up in this book.

There are so many business owners out there with *unhealthy* relationships with this driver, limiting the enjoyment of a good quality of life, and most don't even know it is tied to something more than the need to make some money. They can't work out why, despite saying they're "doing it for the kids", and even when they've given the kids a better life, they're still not happy.

It's why I say *what drives you on can also drive you mad*. It can certainly put a strain on your relationship with yourself and your family if left unchecked. How ironic, given that is what most of us say we're doing it for—the family unit.

From my years of working with entrepreneurs up close and personal, I've observed three very common causes of the pain and self-doubt we're talking about here. Three common reasons why entrepreneurs *really* start their business. Take a quick look and see if you can find one that is closest to your why.

1. A lack of love or attention from a parent (or parents).

This can come about in one of two ways. One is that there genuinely *was* a lack of love or attention from an emotionally absent, violent, or permanently angry parent. The other is a situation where the parent simply wasn't around or was too busy doing their own thing (such as running a business or working all hours to keep food on the table.)

It could even be as simple as being one of many siblings and your parents didn't have as much time for you as you wanted. If you saw your brother getting more attention than you, it can really mess with your head—especially if you're only seven and you don't understand this type of stuff yet. It can lead to all sorts of insecurities and the thinking that the absence of the parents' attention, or the aggressive behavior, is somehow the child's fault.

It's totally messed up in that of course it isn't the child's fault, but it's perceived that way by the child. And perception is all that matters.

It creates huge personal issues that, if left unchecked, stay with you all your life. It means you end up using business success as a surrogate vehicle for your parents' attention and the recognition you crave.

You want to remind them through the success that you are there, you deserve to be noticed, and they were wrong about overlooking you (or treating you so bad). It's as simple as this: a successful business is your attempt at proving them wrong and winning their affection back.

2. A feeling of never being good enough for their parents.

This one is different from the first example in that the parent was there, and the parent *did* give a great deal of love, but it came with an *expectation* of how the child had to live and behave. It had strings attached to it. It was perceived as conditional.

In this scenario, the parent places so much pressure on their child to do well in life that he or she never felt they could live up to the high standards and expectations of the parent.

The love was there, the hugs, the cuddles, and even nice words of encouragement were given, but the child grows up thinking that no matter what they do, they're never quite good enough for the parent. It creates immense self-doubt. The child lives in fear of never being good enough for their parent, no matter what they do, and worry that if they don't do well at school, or in sports, etc., that the love would be withdrawn.

It creates a way of living that means no matter how much success the child goes on to have, they live with a feeling that it's never enough. For anyone.

Their entire life becomes one of trying to live up to their parents' demands and expectations. Cue the never-ending quest to be more and more successful in business and sadly real happiness never shows up, no matter how much money or business success comes their way.

3. Growing up in a house with lots of arguments over a lack of money.

In this scenario, you get to watch your parents' struggle and you see the strain it puts their marriage. It leads to an unhealthy and unhappy household and maybe they divorce because of it.

Years later, you look at your parents and they're still scarred from it. They're still both deeply unhappy.

As you grew up, you got a front row seat to the toxicity and infighting. As a result, you spend your whole life worried about running out of money for fear the same fate will befall you and your family.

It means your pursuit of money isn't for the purpose of enjoying life. No. You want it to make sure nothing goes *wrong* in your life. There's a difference. It's not the actual money you need—it's the psychological safety net you think it automatically brings. You think that if you get it and hold it, you'll never have any of your parents' problems or experience their suffering.

However, because you're perpetually living in fear of never having enough, you're creating new problems of your own.

The biggest being never being happy, no matter how much money you make or get. Worse, it eventually shows up in other areas of your life and means that no matter what you get, you always think you need more. Even love. And that's going to really affect romantic or personal relationships—not just commercial ones.

So What About Me?

As I look at all of these three scenarios, I think I lived for quite some time with the *perception* that I wasn't ever good enough for my parents. Maybe I was, maybe I wasn't. I just *assumed* I wasn't.

@THEPAULGOUGH

Let me explain: I am from a very big family with lots of clever and successful family members around and above me. It was easy to get lost in that type of family and I am much older than my two siblings by ten and twelve years. By the time I was a teenager, they were much cuter than me. It was much easier for people to want to spend time with a happy two- and four-year-old than a stroppy, spotty fourteen-year-old.

My dad and a close cousin were also well known around town for being really good at what they did at work and sport, so most people wanted to know more about them than me.

I was always happy for them both, but I must admit, I did from time to time just wish people asked about *me* and how *I* was when talking to me and not always wanting to know about them *through* me. But I get why they did it. I suspect I often do the same with others.

It also didn't help that my dad disappeared out of my life when I was about 19.

He didn't die or anything like that. He just decided that he had more important things to do than spend time with than me, my sister and brother.

It's funny what that does to your mind—especially as it is still developing and trying to make sense of the world and your place in it. It can make you a little insecure, to say the least. When your dad withdraws love and attention, the person you assumed was here to keep you safe, it can do silly things to you like make you try starting a business thinking that if it's a success, he might give that love and attention back.

Sure, it *might* have done that, however, in my case, the reality was that all my successful business ever did was drive him farther away.

My success probably exposed his issues more than helped mine.

I'm sure he has his reasons for doing a *Houdini* (disappearing act) on us all, it's just that none of them make any sense to me. In forty plus years of being alive and having four children myself, I have yet to find anything that could possibly be *that* important that it's worth sacrificing the relationship with your own children.

Who knows, perhaps he's still working through one of the above three scenarios himself and that's causing the insecurities that he's projecting on to me?

I don't know for sure, but I do have my suspicions.

Anyway, before I write something I might regret (I doubt he will ever read this, but just in case someone he knows does…), the key to all of this is the *awareness* that it's happening to you. It's not to ignore it. It's to accept it. Accept it, then embrace it and harness it.

The real trick is to use all your different motivators at the right time, on the right thing, for the right duration. It's not to get consumed by any one of them thinking that if you are a success then it'll all change and you'll suddenly feel better.

You *might* be right, but it's a massive risk and you'll lose a lot of good days in the meantime. What I'm saying is there's a better way than to spend forty years of your life building a business just to prove someone wrong. And equally, there's better things to do with your money than hoard it hoping all of life's problems will pass you by because you did so.

Roots in The Past

As we come to the end of this very important, and because of that, somewhat lengthy chapter, I want you to remember this, if nothing else: **nearly all of today's unhappiness has roots in the past**. And it's the stuff in your past that will always get in the way of anything good you do in the future. That is unless you go and figure out what it is.

You can't fix an issue with your mother or father by buying a Porsche or making $1,000,000, any more than you can fix an issue with your own insecurity by running a better Facebook ad or building a better email funnel. Something happened in the past that needs resolving. Even if it is just to acknowledge it and accept it, you need to do it.

In that way, you *can* change the past.

Not the actual event, but in the most important way possible, the *meaning* of it.

You may not improve the relationship with your mother or father, but you can change the relationship you have with the *thoughts* you have about it. That makes living your life and enjoying it a lot easier. By applying a different *meaning* to whatever it was, you can move forward even though it happened and, in my case, use it as a positive that propels you to be able to live a care-free kind of life with less angst and less doubt about who you are and why you're here in the first place. Which, by the way, isn't to please others by giving up your own life.

It might be noble, but it's not necessary.

Best, you can get on with running your business and not yourself into the ground trying to make it work at all costs.

When you make peace with the past, and settle on an acceptance that you love your business, and that's why you're doing it, all of a sudden you start to enjoy life it a lot more.

And guess what happens then? Inevitably you will get better at and in doing so make more money from it. On and on it goes. More enjoyment, more money. More money, more enjoyment. It's beautiful.

Thankfully I figured this stuff out early. Admittedly there are still moments when it gets to me, but the thoughts don't consume me anymore. The insecurities still pop up, but I usually just wait for them to go, or I think about something else. And that is usually my early childhood where a lot of good memories of me feeling safe, loved and secure are found.

Anyway, the key point I want to emphasize is that if you're not careful, the reason you started the business can remain an unhealthy driver that controls your life. You can literally drive yourself mad wondering why no one seems to care about your success, or you, or why, despite it all, nothing ever seems to change. You still feel insecure and with a point to prove.

There's no joy from living a life like that.

Discovering what really motivates you—which is unlikely to be money—leads to the contentment and calm in your life you're surely looking for. It means you can get on with building a successful business, making loads of people happy and getting paid handsomely for doing it without a shred of guilt or remorse.

What a beautiful way to live.

It really is worth taking the time to figure out.

Major Principle of Chapter 4: All your pain and frustration has roots in the past and unless you identify them your life will always feel out of control. No matter what you get, you'll always feel like you need more.

ACHIEVEMENT
CHAPTER 5

Why Is Everybody So Serious?

Imagine going through your entire life and forgetting to have fun. Picture getting to the end and being shown the number of days you *really* enjoyed being alive and finding out it's not even in double digits. It sounds like a drab, pointless existence to me. And yet, it's the reality for most. Outside of life events such as weddings, births, vacations, alcohol-fuelled birthday parties, etc., few people find their own excuses to have more fun and live a *lot*.

The typical person's quest for fun usually starts and ends with, "I've had a hard time lately, I *deserve* to have a good time tonight." It means there are fleeting moments of the fun stuff, but it's definitely not a priority. It is a reward, not a way of life.

Sure, there's a bit of pleasure here and there, and even a sprinkle of excitement from time to time. But, for most people, I think it's safe to say that there's not that much genuine *joie de vivre* going on—that is, a delight in simply living your life because you've been given one.

It's a frame of mind that says you *get* to live and enjoy life, not that you *have* to keep finding an excuse to do so.

Sadly, for *most* people, life is usually lived in the vain hope that the struggle will be worth the reward. It's mostly about "hunkering down" and "getting through it," accepting the struggles of life as though there's no other way. It's about struggling hard enough for long enough and if you do it well enough, then someday, one day, Lady Luck might shine down and grant you a release from the prison you're trapped in with all of the other people whose only luck is bad luck.

I get it.

As I said in Chapter 1, I was raised in a small, economically challenged town where many people think like this. Everything is about "getting by" and "being OK" because you "have to be OK." It's about surviving not striving.

I love my town but where I'm from, in Hartlepool, England, everywhere people look they see and hear about a view of life that supports the conclusion they've already come to: that life is supposed to be tough.

Where I'm from, you can exist and struggle, but having a zest for life? That isn't what most people wake up with. That isn't the norm. In fact, they'd think you were weird—or wired—if you did. You'd definitely stand out from the crowd.

But this type of thing isn't just going on in my town.

It's a way of life that many people subscribe to *even if* they appear to be happy when you say hello. For most people, the conversation that they have in private, with themselves, is usually very different from the one you will have when you meet them in the school yard.

It's easy to smile and pretend that life is great when you're out in public, but it's how you feel about life and *yourself* when you are *alone* that exposes the quality of your life.

I don't know if I fully agree with the phrase "Most people live quiet lives of despair," but I suspect there's at least *some* truth to it. The post on Facebook about your great weekend is one thing. But what you are thinking about when you're in the car, alone, on the way home from work and just before you close your eyes to go to sleep are the two situations that reveal how you *really* think about your life and the circumstances of it.

For most, it's not exactly optimistic.

It's also why so many people will say that they hate being alone—they find themselves taking bad advice from an abusive friend who confirms what they lack or are not good at.

Now, this way of living may be common, and is largely accepted as "normal", but what if there was a different view of life you could subscribe to other than it has to be a struggle and taken so seriously?

What if we could turn this around and maybe start to see life a little differently?

As mentioned previously, one of the simplest ways to add real quality to your life—to enhance your enjoyment of life—is to use your unique ability to change what almost everything happening to you *means*.

You and I both have a remarkable ability to dictate the importance of everything that happens to us. It is what makes us different from every other creature on the planet. It means that, at any point in time, we can *actively* choose how we want to interpret what has happened to us and decide how we want to feel about it.

The key point is that we're able to do that of our own *free will*.

If you want to make yourself feel good about something that others choose to make themselves feel bad about, you can. It's not easy, but it *can* be done.

Ultimately, it means we can control how we see life and, most importantly, how we feel about it. And given that most of us decide if we've had a good day based upon how we *feel* about what happened that day, not what *actually* happened, it pays to know ways to change how you interpret it.

This all sounds great so far, but here's the problem: most people aren't ever taught this. Most people know nothing about changing their lives based on how they decide to interpret their circumstances.

Sadly, this is not taught in the school curriculum, nor is it ever likely to be. Playing a *recorder*, using an *abacus*, and learning about *geological science* are much more important for a ten-year-old, apparently.

Automatic Responses

Another problem people have that gets in the way of enjoying life freely is they're mostly told how to react or behave, even before something happens.

Not only are they told from birth that life is going to be "tough," or has to be "hard," immediately altering their perception of the *possibility* of a good and happy life, but they're also conditioned on how to *respond* to life before it's even happened.

What I mean by that is people have been told that if something sad happens, they *have* to cry. They've been told that if there's a political scandal, they *have* to feel angry about it.

We're told that if a parent doesn't love us, we *should* be angry or resentful and feel hurt all our lives. Whatever it is, we're told how we *should* feel about it and crucially, *before* it's even happened. We are *pre-programmed* to feel a certain way about almost everything. It means people have already decided the *night before* how they're going to react to a situation that hasn't yet happened.

And if this is happening, how can anyone claim to be in control of their life when they've already got a response for a situation that hasn't even happened yet?

In essence, what we are is a collection of automatic responses and, sadly, most of those responses aren't positive. There's little if any *independent* thinking going on and so most people's responses aren't necessarily the best one for them, or that situation, at the time.

It's yet another reason why so many people report never feeling in control of their lives. They really aren't. They're responding to their own *unique* life situations in a way that is like everyone else. They *want* to be different and *want* to live differently, but they're all getting the exact same thing simply because they respond to situations in in mostly the same way.

All this is common, to the point where it is accepted as normal.

As normal as not being in control of your own actions and feelings can ever be, that is. But just imagine being able to change how you feel about a situation that you don't like.

How good *could* your life be?

Just how differently *could* you feel?

An easy scenario to explain the difference is to compare how two different business owners see their respective businesses. Let's look at a hypothetical situation that you and I could be in.

If the meaning *you've* attached to your business is that it's something that is meant to be a struggle, that all business owners must struggle, that success has to come at all costs, then your life will become just that—a struggle. You will get what you look for.

However, if I choose to see my business as something that excites and lights me up every day that I go to work, something that allows me to face challenges head on and will help me to learn more about life, myself, and other people, then I will feel very differently about it than you, especially when the same challenges come along.

When a member of staff resigns without notice, sure, it can *really* annoy you.

But you then have a choice. You get to confirm that your view of business is right—that it's always going to be a struggle and that no matter what you do people will always let you down. You *could* do that.

Or you could laugh it off and remind yourself that you *expect* this type of behavior from some people and all that this person has done is confirmed that you should always be on your guard for this type of thing in the future. Tell yourself that although unwanted, it will happen again many times over in your business career, but it won't alter the success of your career in any way. Do that, and you'll feel very different about it all.

And it's the same with life.

You and I both get to decide how we want to see it and feel about ourselves as we live it and that is *in spite* of how other people behave, what they say, or what their expectations of you are. It's not easy, but it is possible (I seem to say that a lot in this book!)

Now, I'm not saying everyone will *automatically* be happier for doing so, but I am saying that more could at least try.

You, Already A Billionaire?

An easy place to start is by waking up and reminding yourself that even if someone offered you a *billion* dollars for your life, you wouldn't take it. In that instant, you confirm to yourself just how valuable you and the life you've got really are.

Congratulations by the way, you're a billionaire!

(Now, what to spend it all on?...)

Another simple way to start your day off on a good foot is to think about three amazing things you did yesterday, as well as consider three amazing things that are coming up in your future. No matter how small, they all count.

They all serve to change your view of the world from one that is all about breaking news, scandal, and inflation, to simple, joyous things that are going on all around you that you might, *just might*, be taking for granted in favor of thinking about the things that have or could go wrong.

Basically, you and I think in pictures. Why not put some nice ones up there to look at? Maybe even create a blockbuster movie that you are the star of and replay it over and over, like a timeless classic that never fails to make you laugh?

Another thing you could do to enjoy life a bit more is to stop thinking that your best life is in the future. A classic mistake entrepreneurs make that is also the cause of most of their angst, I might add. Change the view of your life from one that is all about getting rewards and feeling better in the future to one that accepts that everything you've got *right now* is more than you'll ever need.

To clarify, *don't* do this in a way in which you give up on your ambition and become lazy, accepting what life will throw at you. No, you've already left that world behind a long time ago. Besides, there are too many people doing that already. The world doesn't need any more people waiting for their fortunes to change in front of the TV.

What I mean is do it more in a way that acknowledges that you do want to make progress because that is important in your life, but that same progress doesn't mean *you* will somehow be any better when the progress happens.

Here's a big tip I'd like to share with you: **separate yourself from your accomplishments if you want to feel good about yourself more often.**

You can feel better *because* of the progress you made, but not because of what you *got* because of that progress. The two are very different and massively misunderstood, especially in the entrepreneurial world where accomplishment is often measured by a bank balance or a medal.

You could say it's about *balancing your ambition* with *acceptance of yourself*.

Again, it's not easy. But this is what success at the level I'm talking about in this book is *really* about.

It requires a shift in thinking about how you see life so that you're just as happy today with what you've got as you will be *when* you achieve whatever you achieve in the future. It's not easy, but worth a try. Especially if what you're currently doing isn't working and you're always thinking life will be better "when."

"When I've done this, *then* I'll feel better" is a curse that people put on themselves that can really ruin their enjoyment of life. What is more, "arrival fallacy" is real, and it basically means that no matter what it is, kids excluded, when you get it, it never makes you feel the way you feel

and it never lasts as long.

The trick *isn't* to go and get the next thing, thinking *that* will be different.

It's to change how *you* feel about *yourself* right *now* so that when whatever you're chasing happens, it adds a sprinkle of gratification that is nice, and you'll gladly accept, but it doesn't make you feel better about yourself as you already nailed that piece on your own.

To always think that life will be better in the future is a trick your mind is playing on you. It's likely been saying it for years and yet not much has probably changed, has it? I bet that no matter what you get, the same voice is telling you it isn't enough, but if you go again, then next time it will be.

Sound familiar?

If it does, you're' not alone. It's not just you who is being tricked into thinking that life will get better and I'll feel better *"if I just..."*

I hear it in my own head all the time.

Truth be told, it's possibly the biggest fight I've got in my life. And every day I don't win the fight I risk giving up a guaranteed great today, for the possibility or promise of one in the future.

Now, and as much as it's tempting to live in the future, what if *instead* of thinking the reward for everything you do will come later, you simply looked at it from a different angle? One that was simpler, made more sense, and was easier to enjoy?

For example, what if the reward for living *is* living itself?

What if the reward for a life well lived is a life well lived? What if the *reward* for a life of prioritizing fun and laughter, is, well, a life full of fun and laughter? What if living the type of life you dream of is its own reward?

Why does it always have to be about something else?

Why does everything have to have so many strings attached or consequences and always be about "later"?

If you have one in hand, highlight this next part with your colored marker: *life was never meant to be a struggle.*

Whoever told you it was really didn't get out of the house all that much or was probably in loads of debt buying things they didn't need. Life absolutely is about feeling good about yourself today, right now, and while you do whatever it is you do—not just the end game.

Otherwise, what is the point?

It's gotten so bad that most entrepreneurs care more about the afterlife than the one they've got right now. Their so-called "legacy"—what people think of them when they're dead and gone—seems to occupy their thoughts more than getting the best out of the life they're living today. It's not uncommon for an entrepreneur to spend more time on their estate and succession planning for their business when they're *dead* than living for the enjoyment made possible by a business well run today.

Personally, I've never understood this idea of a "legacy." I find it hard to worry about what others will think of me when I'm dead simply because, well, I'll be dead!

I don't profess to know too much about the afterlife—I've not spoken to anyone who's been—but I suspect I'll not be doing too much worrying when I get there. I am not a fan of worrying about things when I am alive, so I decided it didn't make sense to worry about stuff when I'm dead either.

Sure, I get the legacy thing. But what if the legacy you left was a *life well lived?*

What if, when you're gone, all they can say about you is that you were one of the happiest, most positive people they ever met? That you lived life with a smile on your face every day, appreciating the smallest of things and at the same time working to achieve the biggest of things? That you did whatever it was that you wanted to do, with who you wanted to do it with, unrestricted in how you live your life, blissfully ignorant to the small-minded opinions of others?

What a legacy something like that would be. I think anything else is overrated.

If you're going to leave people, leave them with smiles on their faces any time they think about the life you created for yourself, leave them feeling better about themselves every time they do think about you and, most of all, leave them with a few clues about how to do the same.

Basically, make sure that as you depart, they are all able to agree that you had a really good time. That's sounds like a lower-pressure, more carefree way to exit than worrying over what other people think of you or what you did or didn't do that they might judge you on.

When I'm dying, all I want to be worried about is the fact I'm dying. Why add more pressure to the occasion than you need to?

Tight Suits and Heels So High

As I mentioned earlier, very few people bake fun into their daily lives. Having fun really is something that is underestimated and overlooked in most people's lives. And that's especially true in the entrepreneurial community. Which is why I wanted to bring up the topic of fun in this book. How can anyone possibly say that they have achieved an Extraordinary life if they did it without having fun?

What could possibly be more important?

I believe it's so important that you could say the only thing that should be taken seriously in life is the need to prioritize enjoying it—to loosen up a little and live like you've had one or two alcoholic beverages without having actually done so. *Particularly* at work or in the office, where you spend a third of your life.

The business world can be very *grim* at times. It seems to have invented a code of conduct about what is acceptable behavior in the office and even what you should wear. Much of it could do with an overhaul.

I'd start with getting rid of dark sunglasses being worn indoors and then I'd ban people from wearing those stupid-looking, tight-fitting suits that make it hard for people to sit and impossible to move.

I'd keep the high heels that ladies struggle to walk in, though. They are good for a bit of a laugh! There's nothing funnier than watching a grown adult fighting with her own shoe, having broken it on the way to work. If you ever want proof that people take life too seriously, just watch someone lose it fighting with their own shoe in the middle of the day, in a public place. It never fails to amuse me when it happens.

Seriously, no wonder everyone in the corporate world is so miserable.

Most of them are forced into wearing the same sort of clothes that you would be laid to rest in—a best suit. Every time I see people headed to work in their best suits I often wonder if they got dressed hoping that day would be their *last*. It's as if they are sending the universe a message: "Take me, I am ready, I'm already dressed for it."

Sadly, for many, going to work really is *that* bad.

As for those stupid neckties men are forced to wear, it's no wonder no one is laughing out loud at work. They can barely move their heads and there's probably no blood going to their brains for most of the day because they are tied so tightly. It's hard to have fun when all you can think about is survival.

Seriously, it just goes to show how stupid the world has gotten when people wrap a piece of cloth so tight around their neck that it almost cuts off oxygen to their brain to look intelligent and important.

At the heart of this issue—particularly in the entrepreneurial world—is what seems to be some kind of made-up relationship between seriousness and success. The generally accepted position is that if you want to be successful, then you have to act "professional" and "look it".

Basically, you need to appear miserable and be dressed like you take yourself seriously.

No one really knows how to define that for sure, but if in doubt, pull the tie tighter, stick on the dark sunglasses, and strap on the most uncomfortably fitting suit you can find and hope it does the trick. And maybe, if the mood takes you, the highest pair of high heels that you've got.

Forget about smiling at work and make sure you're not seen laughing indoors. You can do it, but only outside in the cold with the smokers.

Apparently laughing is a sign of weakness these days. It shows that you're not taking yourself seriously and you can't possibly be serious about success if you don't take yourself seriously.

Well...

You could subscribe to that type of life, if you want.

But I for one don't.

In fact, I have just one thing to say on that view of life: it is complete *nonsense*. I *emphatically* disagree with it. I don't even respect it. It's a view of life made up by people who are *struggling* with life.

And any time you see people acting so seriously, you can assume they are struggling to cope with their lives. Don't pander to these people, don't jump when they say so, and, whatever you do, don't fear them. Their seriousness is a disguise for struggle—not power over you.

There's no time for enjoyment in this person's life as all their focus is on making it through the day without breaking down or being exposed. The best you can do is humour them and maybe sympathize with them a bit as they're so consumed with life that they're unable to enjoy it.

Before I go any further, here's the thing I want to clarify: I wholeheartedly believe that you should take your role and your career very seriously. But I think to take *yourself* seriously is a tragedy.

What a waste of a life that is.

If all you do is take *life* seriously, then don't be surprised to find that everything that happens to you always seems to be just as serious. Even the smallest things will be problematic in your eyes.

To someone with a *less*-serious view of life, that person who screwed up in your office was so bad it was almost funny, but to you, it was a situation that consumed you for weeks.

Someone else might view that same customer complaint you got as an opportunity to laugh and giggle with their team about how some people are never happy no matter what you do. But to you, it is the end of the world and signifies the start of the collapse of your business.

Once again, it's all a choice. And the choice is all yours.

You *could* decide to live seriously and take everything to heart, or you *could* look at things from a completely different angle and decide that most of the small stuff isn't worth sweating.

In my humble opinion, nothing is worth spending your entire life walking around like you've just received or are waiting for some bad news. Better to find a big bridge and jump. At least you'll probably make the news and besides, in that way, the bad news can actually be about you and it would even be true this time! It wouldn't be like all that *made-up* bad news that was consuming your every thought.

Anyway, and just to make sure I've gotten my point across, what I'm saying is that you absolutely *should* take your career, your role, or your business very seriously, but you *shouldn't* take *yourself* too seriously. You and your career are two different entities.

I am a huge advocate of taking your role or career seriously, but it cannot come at the expense of forgetting who you really are and why you are trying to be rich and successful in the first place—which is probably to have more fun and enjoy life.

@THEPAULGOUGH

With that in mind, if you take nothing else from this book, I wish it to be this:

You don't have to be rich to regularly laugh out loud.

What is more, chances are that if you start taking *life* a little less seriously, while simultaneously committing to your work and working on yourself, you will get closer to the outcome you want faster: happy *and* loaded.

"Seriously loaded and incredibly happy" is a status available to anyone who is willing to do what is required to get it. Why not make it your number one goal?

I believe that there's nothing more important in your life than having some fun—ideally lots of it —and to do that you've got to make the sound of laughter the norm.

In my house, I make fun a priority. I would go so far as to tell my kids that if they're not living in a house filled with laughter, get the heck out. Start the car and don't worry about your clothes. Just go. Give the neighbors a good laugh as you speed off naked.

As they grow up, I will tell every one of my kids to be *ruthless* in demanding this for themselves. Insist on making it non-negotiable. No self-respecting person would ever tolerate being with someone or hanging around anyone that doesn't want to enjoy life. There's no valid excuse for it and no amount of money or success will ever make up for a life lived with someone who takes it so seriously they worry more than they giggle.

And by the way, there's not a single thing you can do to change someone who is miserable by default. It's neither your responsibility nor is it even possible that you could ever change them.

GET YOUR ACHIEVEMENT BOOK RESOURCE KIT: **WWW.EXABOOK.COM/FREE**

Sure, you can make them smile or laugh from time to time but that's *not the same* as someone making a commitment to themselves to be happy and live playfully on a day-to-day basis.

Here's the headline: anyone who needs someone else to make them happy *isn't a happy person.* They want to be made happy and don't know how to do it for themselves. They're a drug addict looking for a dealer. And that relationship never ends well.

My message to my kids is to be careful of ever thinking that you're *that* good or *that* special that you can make miserable people happy in the long term. You can't. Your energy is best spent looking for someone who is already fundamentally happy and optimistic about life and doesn't take it too seriously—and making that person happi*er* by being togeth*er.*

Remember this: life isn't a dress rehearsal. This is the one and only performance of the night. There's no replay. Live it like your life depends on it.

How Many False Responsibilities Are You Carrying?

It's so sad when you think about it, and yet, this taking of life too seriously is so common.

So why does this happen?

Why do so many people walk through life as though they've just received some bad news or are waiting for it? This one is hard to explain and just as hard to accept. You might need to read it a few times.

@THEPAULGOUGH

Here it is: **an absence of fun in life suggests a big problem with responsibilities**. To be more specific, *false* responsibilities that someone has taken it upon himself to own.

Let me explain in more detail:

The real cause of a lack of fun in someone's life is a *deep-rooted false belief* about how they or other people must behave in life. It's no one else's fault. Not the job, not the person they're living with, or even the pressure of expectation from parents. They live with a *false* sense of importance, leading to an acceptance of all sorts of made-up responsibilities that are equally just as false and limiting.

You've probably heard the expression, "I feel like I am carrying the weight of the world on my shoulders." It's usually said by people who are having a hard time dealing with life. Over the years they've accumulated so many responsibilities that eventually they are being weighed down to the point that they're more focused on the pressure than enjoying life.

When you're feeling "heavy" or "weighed down," it's hard to enjoy life. It makes you tired and when you're tired all you can focus on is how tired you are. It's just how it works. This is why so many people struggle to live playfully or light-heartedly. You can't take things lightly if you're always feeling heavy or burdened. You can try carrying the weight of the world on your shoulders for a while but in the end you will collapse. No matter how big those shoulders are.

The real problem is this: **people think the responsibilities they carry are real and that they must accept them all.**

Whether it is a responsibility for *someone else's happiness* or the feeling that unless you always *worry about tomorrow* nothing will turn out right, people have latched on to all sorts of *made-up* responsibilities that are getting in the way of living life more vibrantly. What is worse, they've been passed from generation to generation with each one gleefully accepting them as though there's no other way to live.

Here, let's look at them more closely.

Responsible for being in control of *everything*.

In the entrepreneurial world, nothing is more tempting (and common) than to think you need to control everything and everyone, and that the only way to be happy and content is if everything is under your command.

And yet, the truth is, it's the exact opposite.

The fact is the only way to ever be in control is to give it all away. More specifically, to give it away and be OK with whatever happens next. *Not* in a reckless way that is more like abdicating, but in a way that recognizes this one simple fact: growth and control are inversely proportional. They work in opposite directions. *You can't grow if you can't let go*.

The day you feel in control is the day you realize that you can deal with all the stupid stuff people do and be OK with it, regardless.

Until then, you're living in a self-imposed pressure cooker, always needing everything to go right and thinking only you can make that happen. The penalty for thinking that way is a life of trouble and stress where even if things did go right, the result wasn't worth what you had to give up to get it.

I found the best way to live is to cut the cord on feeling like you need to know everything or be involved in everything. Instead, limit it to the big decisions that will make the real difference. Let everyone else do everything else. Just work on being able to deal with it if you don't like the outcome or consequences of what they do. Call upon a bit of that self-assurance we spoke about in Chapter 3.

Responsibility for everyone's happiness.

Living your life feeling responsible for everyone else's happiness is another classic false responsibility that an entrepreneur claims.

If you think that your family needs you, and only you, for everything, or that all your employees are somehow dependent upon you and only you, again, you've invented a scenario that suits only one thing—your ego. The ego that says you are *that* important that you and only you can make people happy.

Although I get it, and of course it's another one of those things that is admirable, it is not strictly true and you don't want it to be either.

If you *really* want the *best* for people, teach them to be OK without you. Set them free. Promote an environment at home and in the office that allows people to believe that they can succeed with *and* without you. Give them a chance to believe in themselves and be successful independent of you. I believe it's the greatest thing you can do for anyone.

To really help someone, sometimes you must help them *less*. Otherwise what do they become? *Helpless.*

Responsibility for worrying about everything so that it doesn't go wrong.

@THEPAULGOUGH

As for living life worrying that it is always going to go wrong unless you worry about it, well, here's a news flash: it already *did* go wrong if you live like that.

It's amazing to think this is possible, but if anyone *seriously* thinks they can somehow alter the sequence of life's events by worrying about them, well, I'd love to meet that person as they must have some kind of divine power that has been granted upon them that the rest of us are missing.

Anyway, here's the reality check: the fact is that people have been worrying *so much* over the last however many hundreds of years that if it were as simple as worrying *about the future*, then every generation for the next 500 years can all expect to live a trouble-free life. All the worrying can stop, your ancestors have done it all for you.

From now on, because of their sleepless nights, you can sleep worry free knowing that every car coming towards at 70 mph you will have the very best breaks, and that your mortgage interest rate will only ever go down.

As the lyrics of the song go, "You can worry, but know that worrying is as effective as trying to solve an algebra equation by chewing bubble-gum."

Seriously, there really isn't anything good to come out of worrying in a negative way and most people know it. What it exposes is how little control people have over their own minds and how easy it is to justify that worry as if it's a good thing.

"I'm a worrier" is a label that people love to give themselves, but it also limits them. I get it. But if you've got a choice to be anything in this life, why would you choose to be a "worrier"?

"I'm Not That Important"

So there you go, just three false responsibilities people carry with them. And mostly to no avail. As harsh as it sounds, I *don't* want to be responsible for *any* of these things. It's not a healthy way to live, it's not needed, and it's definitely not the best thing I can do for myself, or the people close to me, for all of the reasons outlined above.

In case you're interested in dropping a few of these false responsibilities, I've found a really simple way to rid myself of those responsibilities that I'd like to share with you. I simply remind myself of the following every single day:

"I am not that important, nor do I want to be."

Seriously, tell yourself every day, *"I'm not so important that I should try to control everything. I am not so important that I should worry for everyone and I'm not so important that I'm responsible for other people's happiness."*

You are special in your own unique, individual way. Claim *that*. But do not try to be all that important. It'll put an untold amount of pressure on your life and create restrictions that will limit anything you can do or anywhere you can go.

If in doubt, drop the dead weight of responsibilities and let others do what *they* should and that is take responsibility for *their own lives and their own success*. Be there to support them if they need it, but don't take on all that responsibility for them.

In the long run, where it really matters, you won't help them like you think you are.

Major Principle of Chapter 5: Holding on to false responsibilities hinders your chances of enjoying your life. Locate them and drop them.

PART 2

ACHIEVEMENT
CHAPTER 6

Five-Star Qualities

This is a book written for entrepreneurs. It's about how entrepreneurs can achieve more in life and business. To do that, it helps to understand more about the qualities that will make you more likely to transition to that next level of success. The journey that you are on as an entrepreneur is as much about understanding yourself as it is playing by the rules of successful entrepreneurship, and the latter has a very distinct set of traits and habits—qualities—you need.

With that in mind, let's look together at what those qualities could be.

Personally, I don't believe that there's any such a thing as a the "perfect entrepreneur" —we all think differently about things such as time, hiring, managing money, or problem solving. However, all extraordinarily successful entrepreneurs have a specific set of traits that give them the advantage over the ones struggling to keep up. It's been my observation that you need six specific traits.

GET YOUR ACHIEVEMENT BOOK RESOURCE KIT: WWW.EXABOOK.COM/FREE

The most obvious that *almost* goes without mentioning is creativity.

Creativity is the magic sauce that all successful entrepreneurs typically have in plenty, and it is also the reason the company gets off the ground in the first place. The ability to see things and create things from nothing is the launch capital most of us rely on in the early days of business. We don't always have money at first, but we have imagination in abundance and that allows us to make things happen even with limited resources.

As much as this creative quality is vital, it's not the only thing that you need.

If it were, all entrepreneurs would be successful. But they're not, are they? That's why you need something else layered on top of creativity. I believe there are five more qualities you need. I think you can get by on three or four of these, but to really make it—to get to the next level of success you aspire to—you will need to have a healthy dose of all five. Let's look at them more closely in no particular order:

1. Focus

I knew that the ability to focus was important, but I always confused it with concentration. To concentrate on a task such as reading a book or finishing an essay in school is one thing. But to be able to achieve your bigger life goals, that are often years in the making, is something different altogether.

If concentration is the battle, focus is the war. Concentration, or attention, is also temporary. You can't concentrate for years at a time. It just isn't possible. There is always something that will break your concentration and although it is useful for day-to-day situations you are in, such as working on a marketing campaign or hiring ad, if you want to make a big impact you must be able to maintain your focus for long periods of time.

Big results—the kind that entrepreneurs like you and I are chasing—come from a *sustained* commitment to the dream. That is only possible if you've got the ability to focus. It's easy to think up something wonderful that *might* happen in the future—as I said earlier, creativity is the hallmark of all entrepreneurs—but the ones who can make it come to life have a special ability to focus on it and actually make it happen.

Facebook, TV, and other people's opinions are common examples of everyday things that can cause you to lose your concentration and steal your attention. But none of these things will cause a permanent loss of focus on what it is you really want to achieve. Only fear and doubt will do that. These two cousins are a potent combination and largely responsible for throttling many an entrepreneur's good intentions.

People tend to think it's fear that stops them.

But it's not.

The truth is that when fear creeps in you *begin* to lose your focus. But it's only when doubt creeps in that you lose your focus completely. The two are very different. Fear is primal. It's always with you. It keeps you safe and it's something you never really shake. It can show up in your life without any warning but if you let it, it will pass.

Doubt is something very different. Doubt disguises itself as fear and when it does it completely takes over your thoughts. And as soon as it does, everything comes to a screeching halt. That's when you'll lose your focus completely and it happens from continually thinking about one of two things:

@THEPAULGOUGH

1. **Whether you are even *good enough* to do what you say you want to do.** Are you capable? Do you have what it takes? Will people say bad things if what you are doing is not very good?

2. **If you're even doing the *right* thing.** Is this the best use of your time? Should you be doing something else that is more important? Is this the type of thing someone like you should be attempting?

Look at any situation in your life. When you *started* to have doubts about what you were doing, I bet one, if not both, of these scenarios played out.

The problem with doubt is that it creates a *hypnotic rhythm* that is almost impossible to shake off—unless you're aware it's happening. Doubt causes you to run these two thoughts (and questions) around in your head every minute of every day and because you don't like the answer you get, you ask it again (and again, and again!) but you never get a good answer. So on and on you go. Stopped from what you're doing while you search for a better answer.

Doubt creates confusion in your thoughts and that leads to conflict in your mind. And it's when you're conflicted that you look for anything else to do except what you know you should be doing—the real work required of your vision. You will know it as procrastinating, and you'll know you've been gripped by it because you will start to do trivial, unimportant things just so you can avoid the displeasure it creates.

Everyone has what I call their "clean the house" or "make the beds" moment.

It's that thing you do that you *wouldn't* ordinarily choose to do, but at the time, it's a better alternative than doing the work required of your dreams.

Personally, I know that I'm being gripped by doubt any time I look for an ironing board and some recently washed clothes, pretending that they *really* need straightening out.

(What happens to you?)

It's so easy to fall foul of doubt and get stuck there for years. The trick is to remind yourself of the dream and focus back on it. In that way focus becomes a tool you can use. The problem most people have is this: focus does not come naturally, nor does it come easily. It can, though, be developed. It must be. A lack of it is the real reason why people struggle to get stuff done. They don't run out of time, they *let go of focus*. They fall into doubt too easily and that's where their time goes—working out if they're good enough or wondering if there's something else they could be doing.

When you are focused, whatever it is on, it dominates all your thoughts. It's a trancelike state that isn't "win at all costs," it's just "win."

Well, that's how it is for me.

There's no thought about what I might have to give up, or by what means I'm going to get there, or even if it will fail. I only ever think about being there. I can see it in my head so clearly that it already feels real to me.

When focus grips you, it changes how you look. You walk taller and with a heightened level of composure. As for your belief in yourself, that is sky high. When you're focused, nothing bothers you. It bothers everyone else, but not you.

I find that when I'm fully focused, I am never worried—about anything. It's when I know I am in my "zone." There are no thoughts going to what might go wrong, only what it will feel like when it's accomplished. Call me naïve, overly optimistic, hedonistic, or anything else you want, but that's what happens when I'm focused.

If negativity does ever creep into my thinking, it serves only as a reminder to regain my focus. In that way, negativity serves me well. Like guilt, there's good doubt and bad doubt. There's a way to use it and not always be used by it.

2. Intensity

Next on the list of qualities is intensity. All great entrepreneurs are intense, and they work at speeds other people can find intimidating. It's one of the defining qualities that sets them apart from the rest of the world. The "ordinary world" typically likes to operate in second or third gear, but it's the entrepreneurs who likes to start the day in fourth and get to fifth before 9 AM.

I like to tell my new employees that working for me will be intense. I don't hide from it. I tell them it's going to be *intense*—but it's *not* going to be *tense*. There's a massive difference. Tense is when everyone is walking on eggshells, hoping nothing will go wrong.

When it's tense, there's a negative, unhealthy pressure and you are permanently one bad decision or one missed deadline from the boss having another breakdown in front of everyone.

I don't live or work like that.

Nothing is so important in business that I'd live my life permanently tense or rigid.

Far from tense, I prefer *intense*.

If *tense* is about stress and anxiety, *in*tense is about speed and execution.

I get so much done partly because of the prioritizing that I do (more on that in Chapter 7), partly because of the speed at which I operate, and partly because I'm so focused. Add into the mix that I hire talented people to compound all of that (more of that in Chapter 9) and it's a devastating combination that is responsible for so much productivity and success in business.

I think fast, I talk fast, and I work faster. It *is* intense. But why wouldn't it be? I'm only working toward goals that are going to enhance my quality of life, so why do I want to wait?

Besides, there's an excitement to working at speed and knocking off your goals at pace. Just make sure the staff know how you like to work and remind them all to *wear their seatbelts* as it could get a little bumpy on the ride.

The thing to remember—and the point of this book—is that a *non-dual* way of living is available. That means you can be intense *and* you can do it *without* being angst all of the time.

You *can* work intensely and still enjoy your life. It's not a sign that anything is wrong or that something is wrong with you. You're not working fast to try to change how you feel or cover up a hole in your life—you're doing it simply because that's how you prefer to work.

Like I said in the last chapter, why does everything always have to have a reason?

What if you like to work fast—and that's it?

It's not any more difficult to work at pace, either. It requires less effort. There's a natural momentum that you pick up when working at pace that makes it easier to get the work done. In the end, working at pace and getting stuff done at speed becomes the DNA of the company and the people in it take pride in all that they've achieved.

You achieve so much more and that's why great employees hang around—they want to keep on achieving more with you. It's a drug they become addicted to.

3. Tenacity

There might be many reasons not to do something—lack of time, sleep, energy, problems at home, etc.—but the best entrepreneurs always find the *one* single excuse they need to get it done regardless.

"I don't feel great today, but I'll get it done anyway."

"I had some bad news yesterday, but I'll do it anyway."

"I feel like I'm out of my comfort zone, but I'll do it anyway."

"I didn't get a good night's sleep and I'm tired, but I'll do it anyway."

These are just a few examples of how the highest-achieving entrepreneurs will speak to *themselves*. The hallmark is that although there are many occasions when they don't feel what you might call "prime time," it doesn't matter. They get stuff done regardless.

I believe most people are more than capable of doing things that they set their minds to. **The problem is that they'll only do it when they're feeling good about themselves**. If they feel right, and the time is right, the magic happens. They can get it all done and work at the speed of light when all the stars align on that one day of the year.

The question is, what about the other 364 days?

That guy with a headache who has a million things to do in the office before he goes on *vacation* tomorrow, somehow manages to get them all done. He's shown he's capable of working productively even if he doesn't feel great. He *can* do it, just not all the time. He needs a special set of circumstances—like the carrot of going on vacation—that cause him to work regardless of how he feels.

Fine. But when those circumstances are removed, this same person does not have the ability to do it. If it happened on any other day, less than 50% of the work would have gotten done. The highest-achieving entrepreneurs have that special ability to work and get stuff done without needing a reason and despite how they feel.

4. Energy

Why do most people spend their whole lives tired? Why, despite however much sleep they get, do they always think they need more? It's 9 AM and people are already yawning. It's 2 PM, and they're still yawning. The first three coffees didn't work so they line up a fourth.

It's true. No matter how much sleep, how much coffee, how many doughnuts, or how much rest they get, people are always tired. If you don't believe me, if you are around any number of people right now, just watch them for thirty minutes and see how long it takes before they start yawning. There are literally millions of people who are sleepwalking through life. I often wonder how people make it back home alive.

So why does it happen?

Why are there so many sleepwalkers driving cars, running offices, and operating businesses? Well, it's got nothing to do with sleep and everything to do with emotional control. It's not about how much sleep they got. It's the amount of energy they lose when they're awake.

Managing emotions takes work. Doing so makes you tired. That's because almost all your energy—the type that makes you mentally tired and affects your ability to focus and get things done—is primarily lost in fighting how you feel about things. That's why it's rare to see a fifteen-year-old with a real zest for life. It's why you'll rarely see a sixteen-year-old who says much more than "OK" when asked how life is. They're devoid of the energy to make it happen and that's because they spend most of their teenage years learning how to manage their new emotions.

It's *tiring* trying to understand how they feel about new feelings.

And if you're not careful, being an adult is just as tiring.

Especially in a world designed to challenge how you feel about pretty much everything. Gone are the days of quietly getting on with living your own life, doing your own thing, with your own thoughts and beliefs, living true to what you believe is right for you and your family.

These days, if you're not on a 24/7 crusade for social change, you're seen as a "bad" human and if you try to watch a game of football or the Olympics without getting caught up in the politics surrounding it, you're accused of not caring about other people or being irresponsible.

I get it.

But what if I can care in other ways and on this occasion, I just want to watch the game?

Why is *your* way better than my way?

Call me cynical, but this is the world we now live in. It's being 'policed' by people who care more about *being right and proving it* than any change they make in world and lots of energy is going to be lost if you get caught up in it.

Here's the newsflash: people don't need more sleep and they don't need more food. They probably need more exercise to build stamina, but they definitely need to stop spending time on, thinking about, or having emotionally charged opinions about things that are mostly irrelevant and trivial in the first place. That is where they are losing most of their energy. It means by the time it comes to needing some of it to make a big decision or execute on hours of important work, there's nothing left in the gas tank to do it.

The result? It gets put off for another day.

Fine if it only happens once, but for most, this is how they live. Addicted to being right and angry if they're not. Energy is lost to things that won't make any difference to their lives and it becomes a way of living that isn't supportive to entrepreneurial success.

The Fastest Way to Protect Your Energy

So how do you protect your energy? If it's that important, surely that's the question we need to answer. Well, let's start with a reality check on why the world is so absent of it in the first place: most people are *insecure, anxious, and failing more than they are succeeding.*

(Harsh, but at least *somewhat* true.)

@THEPAULGOUGH

And the fastest escape from all of that is to focus on, get angry with, or pass judgement on something or someone else. It's a temporary bandage for the equivalent of a compound fracture. It covers up the issue for a few seconds, but it doesn't work in the end. Getting angry or irate feels so good at the time, but the problem is that it doesn't last, and you use up vital energy in the process. Like all things, it's fine if it's only in moderation, but if you do it too often, you'll make yourself tired.

People always comment on how much energy I have.

They look at me and assume I have a special type of DNA that gives me more of it. I can assure you that I don't. Ironically, both of my parents have underactive thyroids. Both of them rely heavily on medication to maintain a steady amount of energy, so it's highly unlikely that I've inherited something special or unique from either of them in the energy distribution department.

Better than any special DNA inherited, I developed a superior ability to ignore so-called breaking news, giggle at the latest social media meltdowns, and shut out pointless conversations from my life. I don't care much for politics or who is in charge, I'm careful of where I look, mindful about who I talk to (and about what), and I'm aware of what questions I ask or where conversations could lead when I'm involved in one.

If I don't like where the conversation is headed, I'll change it.

For example, "What's good?" is much better than "How are you?"

As the CEO of your company, you are really the "Chief Energy Officer." You set the tempo for the company with how you show up each day. If you are low on energy, it won't be long before the people around you are too. It's why over the years I have worked hard on developing what I believe to be the greatest of all skills required to make it through this life sanely: to *not give a crap* about most things in life.

Because, quite honestly, most things are not worth giving a crap about in the first place.

Detachment from the trivial many is the first step to real autonomy in your life.

It's hard to enjoy life if you're caught up in things that you can't control or change. By definition, you are out of control. It's *yet another* reason why most people say they never feel in control. They're trying to change things they can't ever possibly change. It's why big government doesn't work anymore. They're promising change they can't possibly make.

They're promising change at a *federal* level when the most important change that needs to take place is at the *internal* level. The real change that needs to happen is at the level of how people see and think about *themselves*—their own self-image—and what *they* need to do get what *they* want from their lives.

Living detached isn't easy, but it sure does gives you a distinct advantage over anyone else who isn't. It certainly leaves you with more energy. To get there, I stopped trying to be something or someone for people who would never give me anything back. Not in a selfish way, but in a way that acknowledged that some of the things I was giving my energy to never made any difference, no matter what I did.

I humbly decided to take my energy to someone or somewhere else and get on with being the best version of myself, dedicated to sorting my own house out first, putting myself into a strong and powerful position to help others who are willing to be helped.

I'm very proud of myself for doing it, too. There's not a shred of regret.

It doesn't mean I am *not* a "noble citizen."

It doesn't mean I am *not* socially responsible and it *doesn't* mean I'm a bad human being in any way. Far from it. It means I found the courage to live checked out from worrying about things that are mostly manufactured by the media, caused by government incompetence, or created by those virtuous folks running social media and instead got on with making a real change in my own life first.

Protecting your own thoughts and energy to advance the pursuit your own dreams is not selfish in any way—it is the best way to increase the weight of your own *contribution* in this life.

Besides, how can I possibly look my kids in the eye one day and tell them to look after themselves, to enjoy their lives, to get what they want from life, if I didn't do it myself?

That's why it's so important that you create your *own* blueprint for living this way. It's so you can share it with others who want to do the same.

Don't take any of this the wrong way; I am not suggesting that you shouldn't care about your family or your health. Those things *really* matter. But even caring about someone doesn't automatically mean that you've made a difference to someone's life.

Which is the goal, right?

Sometimes it's possible to care *too much,* to the point you want change for them more than they do for themselves. In that way, you've added to that person's own helplessness. As mentioned in the last chapter, sometimes, to really help someone, you must help them *less.*

5. Resilience

How many times can you get smacked in the face before you stay down? That depends on how *resilient* you are. As an entrepreneur, there's nothing more certain than you will be hit with punch after punch from places and people you didn't expect.

You are a sitting duck for people to let you down, lie to you, cheat, steal from you, hurt you at the hands of their incompetence or greed—and that's before we talk about the trouble you get yourself into from your own *overly optimistic* outlook on everything you do.

As they say, every problem you've got started with a good idea.

To me, an entrepreneur is someone who solves a never-ending parade of problems in pursuit of something so big they'll probably *never* actually achieve it. And to top it off, they'll commit to spending their whole lives doing it. It's why being in business takes serious amounts of courage. And as I say, it takes a lot of scars before you will see a few stars.

The rewards are high, but the lows are often emotionally agonizing.

Stay in business for more than ten years and you'll have more than your fair share of stories of being let down by people who will say one thing when *they need you* but do something completely different when it suits them.

You'll get key staff who will one day tell you that they're in it for the long haul, then one week later hand in their resignation via a text message when you're on vacation with your family. They'll send the resignation by text, email, *and* your Facebook messenger, just to make 100% sure you get it and your vacation is disturbed. You will get suppliers who will let you down; trusted accountants will file tax returns incorrectly, costing you thousands in fines; and there'll be staff who use the company credit card thinking it's their own. It doesn't end there either.

Customers will leave bad reviews simply because you raised the prices in line with inflation. And let's not forget the lowest of the low, staff members who are plotting to leave and start their own businesses, taking your customers (and staff) with them.

Sadly, that's just *some* of the many things that are going to go wrong in business. I need a bottle of wine just thinking about them all, never mind living through them all. As the founder of NIKE, Phil Knight, wrote in his amazing book "*Shoe Dog*", "Business is like a war without bullets".

I couldn't agree more.

So How Do You Develop Resilience?

If resilience is such a critical factor in your success, how do you get some more of it? What's the key to developing the thickest of thick skin?

Well, it's my belief that the best solution is to develop a *love* of the challenges that await. Not in a weird way, where you purposefully go out of your way to attract problems. No, I'm talking about embracing problems when they happen, knowing *full well* they *will* happen. You don't always know what type, how big, or when, but you know something is always going to crop up.

The trick is to commit to tackling challenges in your life head on and if you do that, you'll soon develop an addiction to the feeling that only comes from overcoming them. From winning the battle.

Everything you want is on the other side of the problem you *don't* want. Focus on getting there, not on how you feel about the problem showing up in your life. That is the feeling you must become addicted to: tackling challenges and loving doing so just because of the ecstasy that awaits on the other side.

Resilience is a muscle you must train.

It's a lot like trying to pick up a weight that is currently too heavy for you.

The only way to do that is to have the courage to go to the gym and *start* trying to lift weights that are currently too heavy for you. Pick it up, *struggle*, put it back down. Start all over. Eventually, the muscle develops and you are ready for a bigger weight. In business, the equivalent is to put yourself into situations knowing that they could go wrong, knowing that you're going to get hurt in the process, but doing it anyway.

You can't learn to learn to ride a bike from reading a book.

You've got to get on the thing knowing that to get good at it means you will fall a few times. Just make sure you're wearing a helmet. You can't learn to hire staff if all you do is read the books or listen to the podcasts. You can't live your life always "getting ready" to hire, putting off doing so in case you get it wrong or always worried about how you'll be judged for getting it wrong.

Here's a fact: you *are* going to get hurt in business. Your heart is going to get broken and your stomach will be ripped out on many occasions. You will go to bed feeling low, you will question why you're doing it, and you will get let down more times than you would like. Accept it and remember that it's not just happening to you. This is how it works. Success is not easy, or everyone would be getting some of it. Just take the necessary precautions to limit the downside.

One great thing you could do is get what I call a bit of *positive paranoia* in your life. Spend some time thinking through things that could go wrong and asking what you would do when it happens. Being *ready* for things to go wrong is way more important than thinking you always need to know the solution in case it does.

My best tip for dealing with things that don't go to plan is simple: don't get upset or take any of it *personally*. When stuff inevitably goes wrong, laugh about it and congratulate yourself for being right. It's much more fun. I try very hard not to take any of it personally or seriously and I never take it home with me. Before I leave the office, I make it my *most important* mission to be at peace with whatever it was.

Even if an employee has screwed up big time or a key person has quit at 4:59 PM, it's my most important task to be mentally OK with it all by the time I get home. I never want my kids to know if I've had a good day or bad day in the office. I just had a "day." They're all the same—precious. And besides, my four-year-old couldn't care less if the front desk girl just quit. He just wants to kick a ball outside for an hour and watch Peppa Pig after. Which, every time I think about things like that, reminds me of how simple life really is and should be.

OK, that's enough of the star qualities you're going to need to be a hugely successful entrepreneur. Let's move on to the next chapter, where we will explore every business owner's nemesis – or biggest leverage – how they use their time.

Major Principle of Chapter 6: There's a set of skills and attributes that extend beyond a good sales process or marketing plan if you want to make it to the next level. Every one of the six skills and attributes I described can be worked on and improved.

ACHIEVEMENT
CHAPTER 7

Time Poverty

The subject of time—and the role it plays in your success—is undoubtedly one of the most important to discuss in a book like this. That's because when all is said and done, how you use your time is most likely going to be *the* number one factor in what you accomplish in life and how far you go. And yet, no matter how valuable it is, time is one of the most *neglected* resources available on the planet.

It took me years to realize to realize the following: that people's biggest issue is not the actual time it takes to do something. It's the time it takes to get *emotionally* ready to do something. That's where all their time is lost.

A classic example is a business owner who is *always* too busy to hire.

Let's be honest, it takes an hour to write a job ad and place it on Indeed, and then maybe two or three hours to do the necessary interviews. Probably no more than four hours in total. However, it can often take weeks, if not months, for business owners to *feel* ready and actually get around to doing it.

This is what they *really* mean when they say they "don't have the time."

It's that they're taking their time to *feel ready* to do it.

It's never been about the *actual* time to do things, it's the time needed to *feel* ready to get on and do it. And this, I believe, is the ultimate differentiator between the successful and those envious of the successful. High achievers have an ability to speed up how quickly they can be psychologically ready do something and that is the reason why they get so much done. They're not blessed with more time, it's simply that they know how to do things without needing to spend time on getting *emotionally* ready to do so.

Needing time to feel ready is another example of those *automatic responses* that we covered in Chapter 5. People think how they feel is how they *must* feel and that "mulling over" something for weeks on end is just part of the natural process of living life.

Well, it *can* be.

But not if you want to be a high achiever.

Another problem is that most people who are *time poor* hang out with other people who are also just as *time poor*. After all, birds of a feather flock together.

It means they pick up on each other's ways of living and simultaneously reinforce bad habits. As a result, no one ever has any time. Doesn't matter what it is, they never have enough time for it. Observe people more closely, and you'll see it takes them days if not weeks to prepare even for something as simple as one night out at a restaurant with their partner.

GET YOUR ACHIEVEMENT BOOK RESOURCE KIT: WWW.EXABOOK.COM/FREE

They have to feel ready to change their routine, consider what they might wear, what they want to eat, and as for finding a babysitter, well, that's not going to be easy either. Apparently, there's just no one in the entire town with a 17-year-old daughter willing to take $50 in exchange for three hours of watching Netflix with the kids.

Another area you see people loose time is in preparing to travel and go on vacation. I really love talking to people about my travel plans. Especially if it's the night before I am due to fly.

There's often a look of horror on people's faces when I am seated in a bar with them and announce that I am travelling to somewhere like Australia—tomorrow!

The fact that I am in the bar the night before is often enough to cause most people to have a panic attack and that's before they find out I have not even packed my suitcase (that usually tips them over the edge and off their stools completely.)

The question that nearly always follows is ever so predictable, too: "But how can you not be packed?" I respond by telling them I will do it in the morning. I remind them that the flight hasn't left yet, so there's nothing to worry about.

Now they're ready to explode. Their faces are redder than Rudolph's nose and I'm getting ready to call an ambulance if they don't start breathing soon. They simply cannot comprehend how I can be OK about not being ready yet with what, in their eyes, is so little time to go before take-off. And yet, to me, it is perfectly normal.

To put them at ease, I resort to simple arithmetic.

@THEPAULGOUGH

I explain there are at least twelve hours to go before the plane takes off and if I need two more at the bar, and seven in bed, then that leaves me with one hour to put a few shorts and T-shirts into a suitcase before hightailing it off to the airport. *Assuming* I can get an Uber promptly, there's really nothing to worry about.

It's possible that for someone else, going to Australia would consume their thoughts for weeks and months on end. It would take over their life and getting ready for it would be all they would ever think about. That's fine. And perfectly common. The problem is that, in the meantime, nothing else gets done! Everything else stops because this is what they're doing—getting emotionally ready for a trip.

That's why I say time isn't lost in actually doing things, it is lost in getting ready to do things. *It's in getting ready to feel ready to do it.* It's never been anything else. It just takes a lot of personal responsibility to face up to the fact that you *can* find more time in your life if you stop thinking about how you feel about everything and just get on and do the thing.

Difficult in this world, I know, especially when everyone wants you to "feel" your way through it.

This point is similar to what I addressed in previous chapters—people lose momentum when they spend time fighting their feelings. It's why if you're planning on achieving a lot in this life—more than most others—you must master the ability to do things regardless of how you feel about them or how emotionally ready you are. If it's the right thing to do—just do it.

Condition yourself to be able to do things even if you don't feel like it. Don't feel like going to the gym? Go because of that. Go *just because* you don't feel like it so you start to train yourself to do the things you *need* to do, not the things you feel like doing.

If you only ever do things you feel like doing, you probably won't do much other than check social media, order pizza and watch Netflix.

Anyway, one of the best things you can ever do is condition yourself to do things without considering how you feel about it.

If it's on the list, and it's a high-value activity, just get on and get it done. No questions asked. Do that, and soon enough you'll find that more things are getting done and if they're the right things—something we'll come onto in a few moments—life will all of a sudden look a lot different. Good different.

FBI's Most Wanted List

The best observation I've made about time—and one that never fails to make me laugh—is how many people *blame* time for everything that is not going right in their lives.

Most amusing of all is the way the people who say they *never have time* also appear to be the same ones who spend so much time talking about how much time they *don't have*. And it's usually while they're sitting in Starbucks drinking a Frappuccino talking to someone who is also equally as time poor.

Call me cynical, but it's as if the reason for having no time is because they keep wasting time talking about having no time. Who knows? But it's an interesting thought, isn't it?

Let's cut the *BS* and face a harsh reality: the *real* reason people achieve so *little* is because they're always so "busy." Not "good" busy, in a way that they're working on the right thing at the right time to take them to their goals, just busy ticking boxes, shuffling paper, and mostly making sure they look busy to justify their current circumstances.

As the author Tim Ferris said, "busy" is the default mode of the world.

And as I say regularly to my staff, "Ants are busy. But they don't achieve much as far as I can see, so let's not copy them."

Busy is a disease that everyone seems to have caught. What's more, everyone seems to *want* to catch it. It doesn't matter who you speak to or what they do for a living, they're all busy and they're always at it. *Busy being busy.* Ask someone how they are, and they'll most likely tell you, "busy." Ask them what they've been up to, and they'll tell you, "I've been busy". As for why they haven't been in touch recently—of course, it's the same reason. They've been "busy."

It's all fun at this point, but if *you're* doing the same, or you've got more than one member of staff doing this, it's probably costing you a small fortune.

Here's a fun challenge: if you have staff, the next time you walk back into the office where they are working, ask how they are or what they've been up to in your absence. I'll bet they'll say that they're "busy" or "it's busy." One of the two. Ask them anything and they'll tell you, "busy".

And sadly, it's the same with business owners.

Whenever I talk to one who tells me they've "been busy," I know I'm talking to someone who is probably underachieving. They may be working hard, but it doesn't mean they're getting the results they want. I think it's gotten to the point where being busy is a badge of honour that *stressed* business owners love to hang around their necks for everyone to see. It's the ultimate cowbell!

@THEPAULGOUGH

That's fine, and virtuous, and wonderful to spout on social, but remember money doesn't flow to you for being busy, a hard worker, or being at something for a "long time." Money and success flow to those who do the *specific activities* that attract those things.

And yet, as easy as it is to catch the "busy disease," there is undoubtedly someone, somewhere, who looks like you, talks like you, has a similar set of circumstances and resources to you, and yet there they are achieving ten times more than you.

How is that even possible?

How can it be that there's a guy or girl with just as many responsibilities, just as many reasons for why they can't get something done (kids, patients, elderly parents, etc.) and yet, they somehow still manage to get more done?

Well, it certainly isn't because they have more time or that they can somehow magically find more time, as many like to believe. There are 24 hours in the day, no matter what country you live in or how much money you've got.

Many people like to think you can, but the idea that you can find more time, is, frankly, ludicrous. It's one step behind the popular (but wrong) thinking that you can "manage it."

Seriously, thinking you can "manage time" is a bit like saying you can manage the weather. You can manage your people, your thoughts, and your actions all to a certain degree. But you can't manage time. It would probably be easier to manage Donald Trump.

Much like the weather, and Trump, time is immune from criticism.

No matter how much you wish you had more of it; it pays no attention to you. It just keeps ticking by regardless. It doesn't care if you are ahead or are behind, it just keeps marching on. As one of my uncles would often tell me, "Paul, time waits for no one. Best catch some of it while you can."

But the good news is that time, like prosperity, is an equal-opportunity employer. It does not discriminate. If you think it's working against you, it's because of how you use and most likely abuse it.

I believe the best relationship to have with time is not trying to get more of it or manage it. Instead, see it as a practical *tool* that you can use to gauge whether you are ahead or behind of where you said you would be at this point of your life (or business plan).

You can do this right down to asking if you are doing what you thought you would be doing at a given point in the day.

If you are ahead, keep behaving as you are. If you're not, change your behaviour so that it doesn't stay that way. It's that simple. You could argue that time is really a tool for behavior modification.

Instead of trying to manage or manipulate it, I see time simply as a tool for measuring progress against my goals and what I've achieved at this point in my life. That's it. I don't blame it or congratulate it. It doesn't *do* a single thing for me in terms of what I get done. Time isn't responsible for whether I sit down to write this book—even if I have the time to do so. Only I can do that.

That's why looking in the mirror and then blaming yourself for what you did or didn't do with your time is the best first step you can take (if you're not as productive as you want to be).

It's about being personally responsible and pleased with yourself if you *are* making progress, and asking serious questions of yourself if you're not.

GET YOUR ACHIEVEMENT BOOK RESOURCE KIT: **WWW.EXABOOK.COM/FREE**

Personal Pride

A lack of productivity is at the heart of the real problem most people say they have with time. It's not time that is available, it's their productivity levels.

Productivity means doing the right things in the shortest amount of time required to get things done *correctly*. And that is not easy, because it takes *discipline, skill, willpower, prioritization, determination*, and *focus* to do so. None of which come as standard in the human design.

To become more productive, you *don't* have to give up sleep, sacrifice time with friends and family, or need an app or a fancy piece of software to keep you organized, like many people assume. No. You only need the *discipline* to sit and do the work you prioritized in the time you allocated to doing it. What I'm saying is that it requires those dreaded two words that have come up a few times in recent chapters: personal responsibility.

Anyway, I don't profess to be the most productive person on the planet, but I do seem to get a lot done and people do regularly ask me how I do it. With that in mind, let me share with you how I do get so much done.

It starts with *personal pride* and having a *high emotional need to feel successful*.

I like going home at night feeling good about myself and having accomplished things that I said I would. I get a kick out of *that* more than anything I own or money I make. And most other very successful, rich, wealthy, affluent, whatever you want to call them, people feel the same.

That's important for you to know.

The addiction is to *accomplishing* what I say I will, not the results of doing it like so many assume. And really, it's the overarching factor in everything else I am about to say. That's why I wish those rat-bag politicians would stop pandering to the public and trying to make them believe all their issues will go away if someone else pays a bit more tax.

As I said in Chapter 1, the issue that torments most people is how they feel about themselves. And for the most part, what they feel is insecure. They feel unsafe. They feel uneasy about being able to cope with the things life *might* throw at them next. And that doesn't change if someone gives you something for nothing.

What people really want to feel—personal safety included—is achieved only through taking more *personal responsibility*. It is not found in shirking it and expecting others to foot the bill. The more that people feel the need to rely on the system, the less secure they feel in themselves. Ironic, isn't it? It's a system that is designed to protect people, but one that actually makes them feel more vulnerable because of its very existence!

But on and on it goes. People feeling less and less secure, thinking that more free money will fix it for them, getting more angry and violent as they demand more of it.

But as you're seeing, it never works.

Sure, there are a few who really need help. And I love that they get it.

But the other *dozen million* or so sat at home on their backsides waiting for a handout, well, the nicest thing I can say is they really don't know what they're missing out on by *at least* having a go at changing their own lives and not relying on others.

Give me a smaller home that I bought myself than a big one bought by someone else, any day of the week.

Anyway, to give you some background on my life, I have multiple businesses in two different countries, a young family that I love being with, and I really love to travel. I visit at least five different countries per year and that's before I consider the travel I do for work to the different states in the United States.

I employ more than 40 people, I write books, host a top-rated podcast, run big seminars, own 70-plus properties, and I'm responsible for more things than I ever thought possible at this point of my life. Best of all, I am a very happy person, and I don't take many things to heart or life too seriously. I find fun in as many places as I can.

That means I've found a unique combination of being responsible for many things, resulting in making millions of dollars, and yet I am still able to live my life consistent with what I believe to be my true purpose: that is to enjoy my life and simultaneously evolve as a person, husband, father and entrepreneur.

Because I've got so much on my plate, people are quick to assume that I use some fancy piece of technology or an executive assistant to manage my life.

Truth is I don't have either. At some point in my life, I will need an executive assistant to manage my travel, etc., but as I write this book, I am doing it myself.

So how do I manage my life to get the best from the time I've got? I'll tell you, but there's nothing earth shattering about it. You may even be a little underwhelmed by the answer that I could sum it up in one sentence: **My calendar reflects my top priorities and *95%* of the time I execute on the**

things the calendar tells me, no matter how I feel. I wish I could tell you there is more to it, but there's really not.

Here's how my system works—feel free to take from it what you need.

I start each day looking at my calendar and the priorities I've allocated to that day.

Most of these priorities will have been set weeks and months ago. A priority is defined as anything that I deem to have a big impact on my life when I've executed on it. It could be to write a chapter in a book, coaching a staff member, fulfilling a seminar obligation, or writing a job ad and score card to hire a new staff member. All of these activities will add massive value to my life when they're done. These priorities are then put into my calendar well in advance and each one is time blocked.

What I mean by 'time blocked' is that staff calls might be 45 minutes, writing might be two hours, and creating a new scorecard will get about 60 minutes allocated to it, and so on. Everything has a defined amount of time allocated to get it done. What's more, I even put the activities in my calendar at the time of day I know I am in the best frame of mind to do them.

It's not only about doing it, but also about *when* you decide to do them is just as important.

For example, I like to write early in my day. So, book chapters get done in the morning.

And I find that talking to staff or clients energizes me, so I save those things for when I could start to experience that mid-afternoon lull. I'm not immune to it, I just set the day up to avoid it healthily rather than with coffee and donuts. Instead of coffee, I talk to people about things that excite me or keep my energy levels high (business growth being my favorite).

Each day, as I look at my calendar, I have a notepad and pen in my hand that I use to list out all the tasks I need to get done that support the priority I've put in the calendar.

I like using a pen and paper because I like to write ideas next to my priorities and I also like to cross things off. At the end of the day, I can see what I've got done and I can go home knowing I have achieved things that are important to my bigger goals. Doing this helps me feel successful multiple times per day, and if you really focus on that, you get to call yourself successful any time you cross an item off your list.

This is also great for boosting your self-belief.

When you live life knowing you *will* do what you say you will do, it's difficult not to feel good about yourself or be confident in any situation.

If you know you can rely upon yourself to deliver on the promises you make, you really are at a different level of life than most. I've found the trick is to break things up into smaller activities and then condition yourself to be *proud* of the little things you did. You don't need a big gold medal to feel successful. Create your own rules for your own life.

One of mine is that I get to call myself a success by doing what I say I will.

I have even bought my own set of *pom-poms* so that I can cheer for myself every hour or so. Only kidding— although I have considered it!

Anyway, just keep doing it over and over. Keep ticking off the things on the list and never stop telling yourself you did something good. That's all you need to do to keep feeling perpetually successful every day.

I believe that is a much better way to live than waiting for the big applause (the prize) at the end that almost never comes.

Get into a state of mind that acknowledges and congratulates yourself for doing little things consistently well. Before you know it, a lot of little things done well add up to a couple of big things that are then available to you. Money, cars, jets, etc. I think they call them the trappings of success. But don't focus on them. Focus only on what is required of you to one day be in the position to enjoy them.

What's interesting is that I can usually get no more than about five or six things in any one day. I never seem to get to the seventh. Don't ask me why, it just nearly always seems to be that I can get five or six "big" things done each day. And by big, I mean stuff that really matters. Whether it is meeting with staff, talking to clients, writing a marketing piece, or doing some job interviews, it seems that when each item has one to two hours allocated to it, that's what I can get done.

What's more, the most time I can ever seem to commit to one specific thing is about three or four hours. After that, my brain is fried! I'm done with it. I need to be reinspired and to do that I move on to something new to get reenergized, or I even try moving to a new location (such as a library). Sometimes that does the trick.

Like I said earlier in the book, I don't have more energy than the typical person, I just look for things that keep me energized and moving between tasks and environments is one way to do this. When you move rooms or locations you hack the brain into being restimulated and energized by the sight of new things. It's why sitting in your office for 365 days of the year really isn't good for you. It's also why I constantly encourage my clients to get out to seminars and meetings etc., it does you no good whatsoever constantly sitting in the same office no matter what excuse you tell yourself for doing so.

If I don't finish something, I just find a space for it on my calendar the next day and many times I've already done so knowing that a full marketing campaign, for example, might take me about twenty hours.

To clarify, in my calendar you might see five lots of four-hour time blocks with the word "marketing" attached to them with a brief description of what I need to do in that time.

Sometimes it will literally just say "marketing," as it could have been placed there six months beforehand.

I *wouldn't* have known exactly what I would need to do when I put it there, but I know that in my day-to-day role I am required to do the marketing for the company. I know marketing is a top priority, and that it's got to be done—by me—so I'd be foolish to ever arrive at a week without having allocated a time for it.

The most important thing to know is that everything I do links back to a set of key priorities that have usually been established during my businesses' annual plan at the start of the year. And that links to my 3-5 year life plan.

Each day I'll reconfirm that the things I am working on right now will help me to achieve those pre-set priorities I have for my business *and* my life. And doing this is important. Just because it was a good idea six months ago, that doesn't mean it still is today. It means it is very likely to be—but not always. That's why I like to consider if what I am doing is still the right thing to be working on before I get my head into it.

When choosing the things that I'll work on, I'll look for areas that have the biggest impact —you could call them Big-Impact Activities—such as time with my team, marketing, hiring, coaching, investments, writing books, etc.—and I make sure that my day is filled only with those things. I leave a little room in the calendar for things that I don't expect, or for staff just to be able to ask me anything they need help with that day.

In case you're wondering, I don't have an open-door policy by any means, but it's also not so tightly slammed shut I can't get out. I don't want my life to become a military operation where every second is accounted for. That's not how I want to live. It's just a very focused and disciplined one that seems to work for me.

It is a way of staying balanced and centred so that my creativity is maximized without losing the fun and little bit of *weirdness* that I like.

And I am a bit weird.

But aren't all entrepreneurs? We start businesses, take massive risks, not to mention a hammering off the government and the press if we make a success of it, and in doing so have to deal with the unpredictability of employing people. That's weird by any definition.

But as I like to say, it's good, weird. Not creepy weird. Like good guilt, it can serve you well if you use it.

An Entire Hour Looking at My Calendar

On top of all this, something else that I do to help me to stay productive is to spend at least one hour every week looking at my calendar and asking if it is still relevant.

Sounds simple, but it really does help because before you go forward, you should first look back. There's always something to learn if you do.

@THEPAULGOUGH

How I do it is as simple as every Friday afternoon I open my calendar and stare at it. Literally, I just stare it for about an hour.

I look at what I did in the last week so that I can see what I got done and where my time was spent. I then ask myself if that was the best use of my time in relation to my life and business goals.

Essentially, I am asking if my *big-impact activities* are still having a *big impact* on my life—and then consider if I need to re-prioritize anything for the next week. After all, the definition of insanity is doing the same thing over and over, all the time expecting a different result.

Some weeks I spend more in marketing than with sales. Some weeks I am spending too much time with staff and not enough on my own. Some weeks I am doing a lot of recruitment and some weeks I realize I stayed late too many nights in the office.

If that's true, I make a point of making sure I go home a bit earlier the next week to avoid me going out of sync for too long with the family life that is important to me (more on that in the chapter "Balance is Bullshit").

After that, I'll then spend a few minutes looking at the weeks and months ahead so that I'm conscious of what I'm committed to, as well as how much "wiggle room" I've got should something I'm not planning for come up (which it always does!).

I'd go so far as to say this is one of the *healthiest* things I ever do.

I never feel like I am getting blindsided by events or ever going home feeling like I didn't achieve much that week. Simply allocating one hour per week to looking at your calendar can save you hours in doing tasks that weren't necessary as well as remind you of what is important. It's the only practical way to find time that I know of. It also serves as a great way of reminding yourself just how successful you've been.

But, and despite the fact that I think I am pretty productive compared to most, I wish for you to know the following little secret: *I still waste time!* I reckon I still waste about 20 percent of my day on stuff that wasn't productive. And you know what, I don't really care about it either.

After all, I'm only human.

It means sometimes—*many times*—I procrastinate over stuff I know I need to do but don't have the motivation to start doing right away, and sometimes I just do stuff that I think is a good use of time that later turns out not to be.

I am not always highly motivated. Like I mentioned at the start of this chapter, sometimes I am figuring out how I feel about things before I get started.

Some days I feel a bit crappy or just can't be bothered and even though I'll attempt to get it done, it might not be as good, and some days, of course, I've had too much margaritas by the pool the day before (I live in Florida remember!), so it takes me until after lunch to get fired up. I don't beat myself up over this—I just focus on the 80% of time that I did put to good use, knowing that it is better than spending 100% of my time on the wrong things.

Like I said, I do *not* want a life that is run like a military operation. I don't want it to be too rigid. That doesn't sound like fun to me. I do agree that *structure brings freedom*—until it doesn't. There is such a thing as too much structure. Just ask anyone in a corporate job devoid of any room to be creative or spontaneous.

@THEPAULGOUGH

Personally, I value space to breathe and relax, to be at ease with life, in amongst achieving my goals and getting stuff done. I want my life to be less about "I have to" and more about trusting myself to use my best judgment and rely upon the three skills I am constantly honing: discipline, focus, and discernment. The latter being arguably the most important. It is the ability to make the right call about what you need for your life at that moment in time.

My tip is don't spend your whole life deciding today how you will react to things that are in the future and haven't happened yet. A little spontaneity is important in life. You built your business so you could *have more freedom and fun*, not be restricted on what you can do and how you can live. There's not much point to that.

I guess what I am saying to you is this: don't put too much pressure on yourself to use *every single minute* of your life productively. It probably isn't possible, and it probably isn't needed either.

The goal isn't to be so productive that it comes at the cost of being stressed. It's to get the right things done, in an appropriate amount of time, so that you keep moving in the right direction and live *feeling good about yourself* from the sense of purpose that comes from committing to growth and experiencing momentum. Basically, don't overthink it.

Like time management and having a plan, being productive isn't the master—it's the slave. *You* are the master. Being productive is something that *assumes* you'll get more done and have a better life because of it. But it's the *better life* part that's important.

Have the confidence in yourself to give yourself a break on this when you decide you need it and just settle into a simple rhythm of getting the right stuff done.

It starts with prioritizing your tasks, allocating time to do them, and then actually showing up to execute on those tasks—whether you feel good about doing it or not, whether you're feeling on top of your game and motivated or like you've had only an hour's sleep.

Take personal responsibility for what you do, and don't, get done.

Living like this will immediately put you in a league with very few others and in doing so you've already started your ascent to the next level of life where it is so much less crowded and easier to enjoy.

It's fun up here, but there's room for at least one more.

Will I see you soon?

Major Principle of Chapter 7: A lack of time is not the issue. In the end, what you achieve all comes down to the standards, disciplines, and habits that you bring to what you're doing each day.

ACHIEVEMENT
CHAPTER 8

Distractions Delay Progress

As we've just discussed, time might be easy to waste, but have you ever thought about the different ways you *could* use your time? There are numerous different ways you *could* spend time and it pays to be aware of each one.

For example, is it being *invested*? Or, is it being *spent*?

Is it being used *productively* to make meaningful progress towards your goals?

Or, is it wasted because you're *distracted* by things that, although they seem important, do nothing but take your mind off the things that *really* matter?

Although easy to fall in love with, distractions delay progress. You simply can't do big things if you are easily distracted by small things.

I'd go out on a limb and say that most people spend most of their time being distracted from their own lives. Of course, very few will admit to that. And, yes, I know, it sounds a bit strange when I say it. Who would ever live being distracted from their life? I get it. But a closer inspection of the theory reveals the truth. Distractions are everywhere and they come in all sorts of shapes and sizes. They even fit onto your wrist these days...

Maybe you do, maybe you don't, but I still remember the days when time was told by a watch and that was pretty much all it did. It might have had a button to allow it to light up in the dark and if you had a really fancy one, it may have even had a stop clock and timer built into it. But mostly, it just told the time. WOW.

It's an old-fashioned concept and the idea was that you wore a watch on your wrist and would check it from time to time so that, well, you knew what time it was.

The concept is as old as time itself.

And it worked very well.

It allowed you to keep track of the actual time of day and ultimately organize your life according to where you needed to be and when. Wearing something on your wrist, with dials, that ticked every second, was a modest but effective way of staying on track with the things you knew you needed to achieve.

Best, all it needed to keep ticking was a battery that cost a dollar or two and it only needed replacing every couple of years or so.

It was an amazingly simple concept that helped millions of people get to work or school on time, get kids to bed, meet up with friends, and, ultimately, get more things done.

But not anymore.

These days, a watch is the ultimate source of distraction. Far from being a help, it's as much of a hinderance to getting things done. It is the poster child for the type of thing leading many people to the proverbial rabbit hole their lives end up slipping down and with it their ability to finish anything important.

Not content with simply telling the time, these days, a watch will alert you to so much more: it'll actually *ring* to tell you when someone is calling your phone. Imagine that. Life so advanced that a watch can ring to tell you something else is ringing—just in case you didn't hear the other thing ring! And by some technological miracle, it will even let you talk into it.

Assuming you can be bothered to lift your arm, you can now *yell* at your own wrist.

You can literally *talk to the hand.*

Which is another thing I always find quite amusing to witness. For things that give me a good giggle, watching a grown-up yell into his own wrist is right up there with a lady bashing her broken high heel into the floor in the vain hope of fixing it.

As I said in Chapter 5, these things never fail to make me laugh. I don't get out that much, and I never go to comedy clubs, I don't need to. I just watch people do stuff like this. It's all the amusement I need.

But it doesn't stop at a phone call.

These days, your watch will even chime when someone is trying to reach you via text. It'll update you with the latest news headlines, tell you when your favourite soccer team scores a goal, and deliver the "breaking news" that your local politician has been caught in *yet another* sex or financial scandal. As if that type of thing is even news anymore.

It'll send a nudge when someone you sort of know, but probably have never met, has updated her Facebook status to share what she's eating for lunch, right down to reminding you that your *step count* is down or that you need to update your credit card to pay for the next trip to Starbucks that you might have. You know, all really important stuff that you really need to know if you want to make it home alive.

In case the point is missed, let me spell it out: something as modest as a wristwatch is now capable of distracting you from doing things you *should* be doing in favor of things that are utterly pointless and will in no way advance the quality of your life. It's just one of many ways that people are *giving up* their own lives to being more interested in someone else's.

And yet, even though this sounds crazy, especially when you read the reality of just how distracting a watch can be these days, people just have to have one. So much that they'll spend something close to $1,000 on one, not to mention stand in line for *hours* to get the newest version.

People don't have any time, and the reason is they're standing in line for hours to buy something, just to make sure they don't!

For full disclosure, I did try one of these distractions on my wrist. However, I tossed it out the window the minute I realized I needed to carry yet another charger to use it. It was one more thing to think about that I really didn't need to be. When life is at the point you need a charger for the spare charger, you know something is wrong…

But I do get why it works.

These types of watches are a marketer's dream—meaning they're easy to sell—simply because people love to be distracted. That's because, for most people, life is *not* as easy as they would have hoped at this point of it. It's definitely not as fun as they thought it would be.

Most people hate going to work, hate being at work, and struggle to focus on anything negative self-talk and doubt. It's why even *single* people feel like they're in an abusive relationship.

And this is why these distraction watches work so well. Rather than earning a good day's pay for a good day's work, or facing up to doubts and insecurities by looking for a real solution, the wrist beeping acts as a perfect reason to avoid doing any of that good, but hard stuff.

I think some of these watches look really nice. They're a beautiful piece of technology.

But the problem with having so many alerts available at the glance of a wristwatch is that you'll always find something or someone to take your mind off things that really matter.

You'll always skip that project that needs your attention, that book that needs to be written, or that situation with an employee that you know isn't going to end well but needs to be handled.

You'll always find a way to escape work or suppress how you feel. Instead of working through it and developing the self-belief that is missing, you'll instead look to your wrist and find out what your friend ate for dinner to distract you from it. And that is why distractions are so bad. They pull you away from your own life with the promise of someone else's being more interesting.

Why Does Everything Always Feel So Important?

I'm generalizing, but I'm not far off when I say that most people spend their entire lives in what I would describe as *a permanent state of waiting to be distracted from their lives.*

They're not really living life; they're mostly being distracted from it.

How can I say such a thing with so much conviction? Because the average person now spends more than two and a half hours per day on social media. The number is higher for teenagers, it's up to seven hours per day.

And with the greatest respect, you can't seriously believe they're on there learning about how to lead a better life or be better at work. No, they're on there looking at videos of cats getting stuck up a tree or inspecting what their friend is wearing and who they're within the picture they've just posted.

But it's not just an interruption from a watch that can derail your attention.

Whether it is as simple as a noise from the outside, an ice cream van driving past, a light flickering unexpectedly, or an air con unit dripping on the other side of the room, people just can't help themselves from losing control of their own lives by making a big deal out of something that's really quite trivial.

What do I mean by this?

It's this: the next time you're in a meeting, see how long it takes someone to be more interested in the noise coming from the hallway or outside than they are in what you are saying. I bet you can't get through twenty minutes before someone is more interested in the bang from outside than what you're saying about what your business needs.

@THEPAULGOUGH

The problem for most people is they spend their entire lives feeling like *everything* is important. Whatever it is, they think it is *that* important so much they *have* to stop and give it their attention. As if they have absolutely no choice but to give all their attention to this thing rattling outside the room, or whatever it is.

The trick is to realize that the only reason something seems so important is because it is happening to you in the *present moment*. Whatever it is, nothing is as important as the thing you are thinking of, the *moment* you are thinking about it.

It's not the actual "thing"—it's the thinking about it in the present moment that makes it feel so important or so big. That's because anything in your thoughts right now will always feel like it is important. It occupies a special place at the front of your brain and it's consuming your current attention, so of course it feels important.

Whatever you're thinking about in the moment always finds a way to feel bigger than it should be and the hallmark of someone who suffers badly with this is they always, no matter what, make things out to be a bigger deal than they need to be.

I get it.

But it's mostly true that whatever you're thinking about isn't even important *at all*.

Another example of this is the telephone. Specifically, a mobile phone.

It's an item that most people would agree is a vital tool to have if you're running a business. And yes, of course, it is difficult to run a business without a phone. But if you place too much importance on the role of a phone, and specifically, you thinking you always have to answer it, then it'll become a huge productivity drain and limit what you get done.

I realized this many years ago.

It is the reason why I have had my phone on silent ever since. It rings, but I can't hear it. I do not want to be contactable at other people's convenience.

After all, no one is ever calling me for my benefit, are they?

It's nearly always something *they* want or that *they* need to know, in the time *they* need to know it. What I'm saying is when someone calls it rarely ever benefits *you*, does it? I can't recall ever answering the phone to be told by a lawyer that my great-grandad had left me a load of money in his estate.

It's why I decided a long time ago that answering the phone is really overrated. It doesn't make sense to me to do so, especially when someone is willing to do it for $15 per hour.

How far do I go with *not* wanting to be accessible?

Well, a few years back, when I opened my first physical therapy practice, the people from the phone company came to install all the new phone lines. They got to the room that was labelled as "Paul's office." They asked me where I wanted the phone positioned and when they did, I immediately pointed to a desk that was in another room. Where my staff were sitting.

The guy thought I was joking.

But I wasn't.

In fact, I asked him if *he* was joking.

I reminded him that I had a business to run and that if I had a direct phone line in my office, I wouldn't be able to do much of that.

I repeated to him that I paid people to answer the phone for me and that if I did it myself, they were effectively being paid to do nothing. The people I employ aren't expected to do my job, so why would I be expected to do theirs? I told him I have a mobile phone and I'll call people, withholding my number, at pre-arranged times to discuss things that have been decided we'll talk about beforehand.

Radical? Not really. It's just common sense if you ask me.

Being contactable all day every day might make yourself feel important. Which is fine. I get it. People love to think that only *they* can solve everyone's problems. We discussed this in the earlier chapter on *false responsibilities*.

But I'll tell you the same thing now as I did then. The problem with being important is that it also *limits* the quality of your life. It limits the freedom and autonomy in your life, and it also limits how much progress others can ever make if they think that they can only get things done with you around.

Rather than being important, I suggest you focus on being *responsible* for more things. Start with being *responsible* for someone you have hired and trained to answer the phone for you. That way you can move around freely and be more autonomous in your life *without* having to be answering calls or emails from random people while you're getting on a plane to somewhere exotic with your family. It's a much better way to live.

You can still get stuff done, and you can still help people out, but you can do it on your terms, at a time that suits you. Which is the goal of running a business, right?

A Cure For Pointless Emails

If the phone is the queen of distraction, then surely email is the *king* of it. The two are definitely closely related. It's why I have just as much distain for my email account as I do owning a mobile phone. I hate email. Scrap that, I *really* hate email.

To clarify, not the type you send to clients that make money and give them opportunities to buy things from you—those emails I love to write and send.

I mean the ones that people send to you that you feel an obligation to read and to which a reply is expected. The type where you have to spend fifteen minutes reading a load of drivel, about things that are mostly uninspiring and unimportant, to anyone but the sender. It's *those* types of emails I'm talking about; *those* types of emails that even when you spend fifteen minutes replying, always seem to invite another (even longer) email less than an hour later requiring an even longer response.

Which is another thing. Have you noticed how *long* emails are these days? It's as if people *don't have the time* to write short ones.

To counter this nonsense, I've developed a simple little trick of ignoring most emails, depending upon the name of the sender. The ones I choose to look at, I do so quickly by only ever reading the last two paragraphs. That's because it's nearly always in that *last* few hundred words that people eventually say what they couldn't say in the previous 1,000.

Emails really are the worst.

They're a huge time suck for many business owners. Personally, I see receiving an email as another opportunity to have some fun. Sometimes I will reply to a 2,000-word email with something as simple as, "This sounds amazing, let's book a ten-minute call to discuss what you need. Here's my link to book one." Of course, they rarely ever do. That's when I know what they were talking about was pointless.

@THEPAULGOUGH

The other thing I do when I go through a phase of getting too many emails is slap on the "out of office" response saying that I'm unavailable, and often for weeks or months on end.

I tell people if they want something from me in the time I am "away," then they are to contact my office (that I am sitting in), where they can expect to be dealt with promptly by my team (sitting next to me.) Better yet, I ask people not to bother doing that and instead get back to me in a month upon my return from being "out of office."

I often have a bit of fun with the message in my OOO response, too.

Rather than just telling people something boring like "I am on annual leave," I like to tell people I am going to somewhere like Timbuktu for a month, and I don't know if the Wi-Fi there is any good yet, so I can't possibly promise to reply to their emails.

It tests what is really important and what really needs my attention, not to mention who has a *sense of humor* and doesn't.

And in case you were wondering, *no*, as of yet, I've never been asked if I enjoyed Timbuktu. However, I'm certain there'll be a day that I will be asked by some poor soul who takes life ever so seriously they didn't get the joke.

Anyway, I digress.

In nearly two decades of having an email I've concluded that 98% of what I get is irrelevant, so I barely look at it. That's the bottom line. The only good thing about email, if there is one, is that you can make a lot of money if you send enough of the right type, and that you can check it at your convenience. And for me, that is usually no more than once at the start of the day and once at the end.

Where Should You Be Spending Your Time?

We've spoken a lot there about distractions. Being distracted is just one of *four* ways you *could* spend time. Next, let's look at the other *three* ways in which you *could* be spending time and make sure you're spending as much time as possible, in the right way, to have the most fun and make the most money.

1. Tasks

Doing too many tasks is where most entrepreneurs who are stuck, well, *get stuck!* If distractions are "bad," then tasks are marginally better. They are what I would call "busy work." It's usually instantly gratifying and is the type of work that other people can visibly see you are doing, or you can easily explain.

It's also work that makes you feel *less* guilty about the lack of progress you're making.

There's little if any extra income, but you've done a lot lately. There's no money, but you're tired, so that's OK. There are no vacations or time with the kids, but you're working hard, so that's OK. There's lots of hustle and grind, but little in the way of any real progress. That's the hallmark of an entrepreneur's life who is spending time on too many tasks.

This type of activity includes doing things like payroll and accounting, ordering things for the office, booking travel, paperwork, and even dealing with patients or clients. Yes, even dealing with your clients, customers, or patients. This is a task that someone else could—and probably should—be doing for you at a much lower hourly rate than you are worth as the business owner.

Why would any business want to do their own bookkeeping or accounting when you can pay a professional to do it at a much lower rate than you can earn, and likely get it done much better? It baffles me that this would happen, but this is where people spend their time. On tasks.

They defend their choice by saying something like, "But it's only a few hours per month." The problem is they say that about *ten* different things and, in the end, they add up to a full week's worth of a few hours spent on lots of different low-paying tasks.

In my consulting work with physical therapists in private practice, many of them get addicted to seeing patients. They will commit to seeing patients over and above almost anything. To the point where it *costs* most of them money to do so. It's why I tell many they have a *charity* or at best a *job*, but not a viable business.

And when I question further why they would rather see five patients than, for example, spend that same time on a marketing or hiring campaign, their response is that they make "$250 per patient for doing so" (or however much they charge.) They look at the dollar amount, which I agree, is significant, and think they're getting paid well to treat patient, so they continue to do so.

The problem is, treating a patient is not worth $250.

That's because even if the patient is paying $250 per one-hour session, the actual *task* of treating that patient is worth no more than $40-$50.

How so?

Because the hourly wage of any physical therapist capable of treating that same patient is precisely that, $40-$50. The real amount of money being made by treating the patient is a fraction of the total amount received by the business, required to make said business viable.

This also reveals a worrying lack of commercial awareness in anyone who thinks this way.

If Mrs. Smith is arriving at a physical therapy practice for treatment, she may well be paying $250 per hour. But the value of the actual treatment provided is not $250. The treatment cost is just one of the many things that must be considered and built into the fee structure of the business.

For example, what about rent? And how about the utility bills and the cost of getting Mrs. Smith to be a patient in the first place? Marketing isn't free!

The fee to cover the treatment is just one part of why the clinic needs to charge $250 and it's also why attending to customers, patients, or clients, although admirable and gratifying, is really a *low-paying task*.

Now, given that most business owners spend most of their time with clients or patients, it's easy to see why most of them never make that much more than an employee.

But why should they? They are doing the same type of work—tasks.

2. High-payoff work

Spending time doing high-payoff work is where you will *start* to see an increase in your income. It's work that you might not be able to leverage or automate, but it does pay out handsomely at the time.

For example, as much I said that seeing patients is a low-paying task, there'll always be one who wants to pay ten times as much as everyone else that would make seeing them worthwhile.

I haven't treated patients for many years because doing so would cost me money. My time is worth so much more than what I could ever get from *most* patients. However, there's always a price to do so. If a patient wanted to bring me out of my self-imposed early retirement, I would be tempted to do so for, say, $2,000 per hour. And I'd ask for it in cash.

But even then, I'd be looking for a way to get more out of that session by recording it or letting one of my staff watch what I did so they can learn from it and repeat it many times after. In the end, making me a lot more than $2,000.

Other types of high-payoff activities includes things like online webinars, seminars, workshops attended by lots of people, and staff training. It involves business development meetings, especially if it's a sales meeting with a potential customer, a joint venture partner or your team getting together to come up with new sales promotions.

Although important, where possible you want to delegate as much of this work to other people. For example, you should oversee the marketing campaign, but ideally, you're not pressing the button to publish the email or push it out to Facebook. That is a *task* that someone else can do for you. It's still high-payoff though because if the marketing campaign generates $10,000, but you only have to get involved for one hour of the ten, then it was a $10,000 per hour activity. That is high-payoff.

3. High leverage

If high payoff is where your income starts to increase, this is where it begins to explode. When you look back at your week, this is where you want to have spent 80% of your time. It is doing work that is highly leverageable.

So what is a high-leverage activity? It can be explained very simply: it means doing something once and yet you're going to get paid out for it many times over and in multiple different ways—even when you're not there (and even if you are not alive, for that matter.)

That is the litmus test for high-leverage work. It's anything that you do that is still working to make money, even if you are not there, and even if you did it years before. This is the work that really grows your business and ultimately explodes your income. This is the work that is the most rewarding financially and simultaneously gives you back your time even though your business is growing.

This book, for example, is an example of high-leverage work.

Time spent on this doesn't result in an instant high payoff. I won't make loads of money from it all at once, but it is hugely leverageable for me and will pay out in the long run.

I can use it for many years to come to attract new clients for my marketing and coaching business. I can use it for marketing purposes, finding new leads, getting on other people's podcasts or stages to speak to potential customers, and, more than anything, I can leverage the status of being a multiple-time best-selling author. Which, I must admit, is pretty cool.

I can also take some of the content from the books to talk about on podcasts, my team can pull quotes for my social media channels, we can create blogs for the website, and we can even turn chapters of the book into special reports that we can give away in our marketing for lead generation.

@THEPAULGOUGH

Best, I don't have to do any of what I just mentioned. My team can now do their jobs better without me having to get involved. While they do that, I can be doing something else. This is what leverage is about. It is the ability to get more done with the same or less time invested. It is building *on top* of things that you've previously created, that each work without you, while you're simultaneously working on something else that also works without you.

Best, it doesn't only give you *work* leverage; it also offers what you might term *life leverage* too. Because of the type of work you do, it means you have more time take in more places and other fun things. More than most people around you who will be perplexed at how frequently you do so.

When you build leverage into your life, what happens is you end up living the equivalent of multiple lives in comparison to other people's one and only. By that I mean you get to *do* and *experience* so much in such a short period that you do more in five-year life cycles than most do in the entirety of theirs. This is what has happened to me. I've been able to simultaneously run a successful business as well as tick off "bucket list items" and travel to more places, and as I look back on any given year, I've often done more in that year than most people I know would do in ten.

That's why it goes without saying that this is the most important type of work to commit to if you want to raise your income, your choices and quality of life. And yet, it's also the work that most business owners who are *stuck* in the business—doing tasks and being distracted by their staff—can't ever seem to get done.

They'll say they can't get out of the business, but the reality of it is they got stuck by not doing this type of work in the first place.

@THEPAULGOUGH

If a physical therapist is always busy treating patients, it means they can never find time to work on the automated systems, or ever think about a new growth strategy that is different from the one that has currently got the business stuck. There's no time for creating marketing assets or hiring and building the team, it's all *task* type work and as a result there's no leverage anywhere. The income flatlines and so does their excitement for their business. And sometimes, life in general.

It's common, but it doesn't have to be like that.

The first thing you must do is get past the bias or urge to do the work you've always been doing. It's another challenge that you're going to face as a business owner that very few people warn you of. All most people do is tell you about the need to get more clients, not the need to one day stop seeing them. There's no consideration to what you do to make a success of your life, not just your business.

It's not easy, but when you commit to doing this type of work and making it your default setting, eventually you will find that your lifestyle is funded by money coming in from places and activities that you can't even remember working on.

You'll walk into the office and another client has arrived from an automated email funnel you wrote five years ago, and then another from a book you wrote six years ago. You just cashed one check and then you find you must face the "hardship" of going back to the same bank to cash another check you just received for something else you got paid on for work you did a year ago.

Of course, there's no hardship in it all. Cashing checks is a sheer delight. One of life's greatest little pleasures. I hope the government fails in its bid to make everyone use a credit card. Walking to the bank to cash cheques will never grow old on me. It might not be the best use of my time, but it sure makes me happy.

Anyway, if you pushed me, I'd say that any form of automated marketing, follow up funnels, or marketing asset creation is the best form of high-leverage activity that you can do.

The best thing about creating and having these types of marketing funnels for your business, especially if powered by a software like *PhysioFunnels* (www.physiofunnels.com) is that your returns are exponential and the results keep coming in years later.

It means while you are on holiday, leads are converting to paying clients. You're making money and you're not even in the country.

Isn't that the dream?

Well, that's precisely how I grew my first business. I moved from chasing doctors and dealing inside of the insurance system to creating marketing assets and funnels that worked for me, 24/7, long after I created them.

But it's not just marketing.

High-leverage work also involves any form of staff training that is ideally recorded, team meetings run well—that means with an agenda—and it definitely includes quarterly and annual planning. Growing your team and giving them more skills to do better work for you, especially in a group setting, is easily one of the best uses of your time.

And don't worry that they'll get so good they'll leave. Better that than be so *bad* they can only stay with you because no one else will have them.

Anything to do with hiring and recruitment is also included in this type of work class. After all, people are your most leverageable asset. Your time could be spent improving the interview process, the hiring funnel (you can automate that too), or job ads, and even the onboarding process.

Ideally, you're spending your time showing someone else how to recruit and hire for you, using "your style" so that they know precisely how to find the talent you need to grow. You work with one person, and they find thirty talented people over the next few years. In exchange for the time you invested in training just one person, it's possible to build an entire team.

That is high leverage at its very best.

There's nothing magical about high-leverage work—it's just getting over the fact that you don't immediately get paid out when you do it like you might with tasks. It's a mindset thing.

Everyone around you, who ironically probably isn't rich, will likely tell you the key to getting rich is to "work hard." But it's not. There's more to it. There are a lot of people who work hard with nothing to show for it. The secret is to work hard on the *right things*. That is what this chapter has been all about and now that I've introduced you to the subject of leverage, go ahead turn the page and let's look at it in even more depth.

Major Principle of Chapter 8: Move on from doing tasks if you want to make more money and have more free time.

ACHIEVEMENT
CHAPTER 9

Rough Diamonds

I always say that whatever level you are at in business right now, it reflects the level of the people you've got inside that business. What is more, it also exposes the level of commitment you've made to them. If you're doing "OK," your people are probably "OK." And equally, if your business is world class, your people are probably world class too.

It's very difficult for anyone to achieve anything in this world without getting good—very good—at finding other people to help do it.

Eventually, no matter how good you are at what you do, or how hard you work, you can't get past the production that you alone are capable of. It's not possible to multiply your income by ten times just by working ten times harder. There wouldn't be enough hours in the day. It's why you need to make use of the ultimate leverage available to you in life—other people's time and skills.

The idea that we need good people to grow a company is not new.

It's a universal law of business that you need good people to grow a good business. And yet, that's not how most business owners think. On the one hand, they *know* they need good people. On the other, there's always something more important to do. There's a contradiction between what most think and what they do and because of that, there's often a struggle to grow beyond what the owner can do by him or herself.

One of the primary reasons that business owners will tell you they don't hire is because they don't have time for it. As discussed earlier, they always think it takes longer than it actually does but that is mostly because they're getting "ready" to do it.

Ironically, one of the other reasons they are too busy to hire happens because they're always too busy doing something the person they need to hire should be doing for them.

Remember this next sentence: The ultimate sign that you need to hire is being too busy to hire.

The other, less obvious, reason they don't hire is that most business owners have an *identity* of who they are and this identity often limits what they can realistically achieve.

Let me explain:

Most business owners, when thinking about who they are, do so through the lens of a "doer," always "doing" the thing they "do."

For example, years after qualifying as a physical therapist, it's common that the owner of a physical therapy clinic still thinks of himself as a "physical therapist." That is the thing they "do" and that is what they focus on when trying to make money or grow the business.

The theory is that if they "do" more "doing"—that is, seeing more patients—then the business will grow. And it works, at first. But only to a point. And that point is when there's no more time in the day to do any more "doing." And when that happens, there's no more money to be made and no more personal growth to be found.

This was something I had to learn for myself.

I had to come to the realization that my identity—who I *thought* I was—was out of date and holding me back from getting to the next level of my life.

I started my career as a physical therapist and when I realized I couldn't be a professional soccer player, it was all I ever wanted to do. It was in my mind from about the age of fourteen. I went on to have a great career that involved being a physical therapist for two professional soccer teams in the UK, as well as owning my own very successful private practice. It was amazing and I loved doing both. I proudly thought of myself as a physical therapist and any time anyone would ask what I *did*, I'd reply confidently, "I'm a physical therapist."

It made sense to do so because that's what I "did."

However, thinking that way massively *limited* what I could achieve.

Even if I was *the world's best* physical therapist, I knew there would be a ceiling to what I could earn, and my life would always be limited by the need to be inside of a treatment room. After all, patients don't treat themselves. If I wanted to get paid, it would have to be me *doing* that and *doing it* every single day. I faced the prospect of living my life always *doing* the things I'd always being *doing*.

Fine.

But to grow, to get to a new level fast, I had to stop thinking about being a physical therapist—even becoming the best one ever—and instead start thinking of myself as something completely different. What I needed to do was to see myself *not* as a great physical therapist but instead as a builder of great physical therapy *teams*.

Can you see the difference?

One involved me trying to do everything on my own, which has a limit. The other involves finding others to help me do it, which has almost zero limits. My potential is *exponential* as a team builder.

I often say that my business life has experienced *two* big shifts.

The first being the day that I moved from thinking of myself as a physical therapist to thinking of myself as a *marketer* of a physical therapy service. The ability to find clients is way more valuable than serving them and it showed in the money I made.

However, the second and easily the biggest shift, the day my income and the autonomy in my life *really* exploded, was the day I started to think of myself as a "talent spotter" and a "team builder."

Getting good at talent spotting—finding great people—and building great teams has changed the circumstances of my life completely.

It's allowed me to find more freedom in my life to work on what I want, to live and be in almost any place I want, and all without having to explain anything to anyone. Most days my own mother wouldn't know what country I am in. I've engineered my life so that I'm the *least important* cog in almost every wheel of my business—except for marketing—and I let people get on with running those wheels for me instead.

Sure, I am still responsible for it all—and lots of people to boot—but I can be responsible from anywhere and any time zone I choose. Which is precisely how I like it. I love waking up in different time zones and the reason I can do it so frequently is because of the *good* responsibility I have claimed and owned to hire and manage people.

All the freedom I've got, not to mention the money I make today, is found in the leverage I get from hiring great people. It's why I say the secret to getting ahead in business—and in life in general—is leverage.

The Ultimate Leverage

The problem is that, trying to do it on their own, most people simply can't work hard enough for long enough to keep up fast enough with the financial needs of a good life.

It isn't that there's not enough money around, there's more than ever. The real issue is trying to do whatever it is you're doing and doing it yourself.

The reality is there's not enough work you can ever do *on your own* to get ahead for long enough before the inevitable expenses of life start racking up.

You need leverage to get ahead in life. And other people's time and skills are the *ultimate leverage*. When you have multiple people involved, you get more things done in less time, you can create multiple streams of income and you can make a good bit of money before life's inevitable temptations catch up.

And by temptations, I mean things and stuff, cars and houses, watches and clothes, TVs and sofas, weekends away and vacations in nice places. These are the things people get caught up in and struggle to keep pace with.

Far from being a hassle or necessary evil, hiring people and leveraging their time and skills is the key to extraordinary success in business *and* incredible experiences in your personal life.

Being a team builder opens up endless possibilities for what you could achieve and what you could experience. It definitely trumps going to the office to do the same *task* day in and day out. Even better, the impact you could have really could be ten times more because you've now got multiple people involved in the goal.

If you love helping people, you can help ten times more.

No matter how good you or I think we are, there's no getting away from the fact that hiring ten of the right people could do a lot more than you ever could on your own.

Even if they work at 80 percent of the level you do, ten times 80 percent (of what you do) is a lot more *impact* than you could ever possibly achieve on your own. All you need to do is find the right people, put them into the right company structure, and make sure they all know what you want them to do.

Hiring the right people and putting them into the right structure that encourages great communication is, I believe, the real key to success in business. Whenever you see a business really start to grow, and continue to do so, it's because this is where the owner's focus went: on people, structure, and communication.

If you commit to becoming a world-class team builder, or even just being better at it than you are now, the success that you are capable of really is limitless. In the mastermind program and coaching that I do with other business owners, this is what we obsess over; helping great practitioners become better business owners by becoming better team builders.

Sure, you must accept a few more responsibilities and there's a little more pressure. But don't forget, much like good guilt and bad guilt, good debt and bad debt, there's also *good* pressure and *bad* pressure. I think it's better to pick one than be burdened with one. The pressure of managing people is a good pressure if you ask me. It's a privilege. It's positive pressure that is worth it.

And what is *bad* pressure?

It's the type of pressure that comes from never having enough money or ever being able to spend quality time with your kids. It's pressure that comes from always worrying about having enough to cover your bills. It's pressure than comes from knowing you've got a limited amount of time on earth and you're not living it how you would like.

That's real pressure.

It's *negative* pressure and it's not healthy to live with it.

"Find Me Another Rough Diamond"

If you want proof that getting good at hiring people is a worthwhile commitment, just go and study unsuccessful, unhappy, usually stressed out, and mostly time-poor business owners. They all have one thing in common: a *bad attitude* when it comes to their staff (or people in general). There's nearly always a moderate to severe level of *contempt* toward the importance of getting the people thing right.

The *unhappy* business owners are usually the ones who, no matter what, never have a good word to say about any of their staff. It's always some sob story about how their staff can't be trusted, how they don't care enough, or aren't smart enough. And this despite the fact all these people were hired by the same business owner telling the story. Talk about self-imposed misery!

On the flip side, you can also just as easily spot the *happiest* and *richest* business owners in the room as they're the ones talking positively about their team and people in general.

There's a reason they say *culture eats strategy for breakfast.*

It's because you can have the best business plan, but if you don't have the right people to execute it for you, then it's pointless. You'll just end up with a hot mess of a business that is more about high drama than high performance. However, the best people working on a strategy that is even half decent will likely produce significantly better results.

Personally, I think the first place people in business must make a change, if they want to see an improvement in their results, is in how they value the people on their teams.

An easy place to start would be to view people as assets, not expenses.

Accountants and CPAs, who are mostly *useless* at running a real business by the way, traditionally refer to employees as "expenses." But they're not. They're actually *highly leverageable assets*. If hired and trained correctly, and if communicated with regularly, people really can be wonderful assets to a company, allowing it to grow fast. In fact, there's no other way to grow.

As I write this chapter, I have more than forty staff hired from all over the world.

That's a lot to some people.

But guess what I also have? Lots more free time.

I take more time off these days than I ever did when I was a solo physical therapist or even a fledgling practice owner with only a handful of staff. It's why I would tell anyone growing a business that if there's any single reason to commit to building a bigger business, it's that the bigger it gets, the less demanding it is on your time. If you're doing it right, that is.

And of course, only to a point. There is a point of diminished returns as you grow where what you must be responsible for won't be worth what you get back.

In my experience, the worst type of team is a *small* team. That's because everyone is so reliant upon each other that it creates an unhealthy pressure that sometimes makes it difficult to enjoy.

Sure, you *think* it's easier to manage because there are fewer people.

On paper, it makes sense.

But is it really? When one person is off on a five-person team, the others are dragged all over trying to cover. It's a nightmare. However, if one person is off on a twenty-person team, everyone just thinks that person is on the toilet longer than normal, working from home, has COVID (again!), needs to visit the vet, their car broke down, or something else like that.

Basically, the business owner doesn't even hear about it.

This is important for you to understand.

If you're after material success—money, holidays, houses, etc. —then having the right people around you will make that happen faster.

And, equally, if you're after more lifestyle riches, that is more time for yourself or with family, even just to stop doing some things that maybe you don't like to do and do more things you love to do, then having the right people around you will make that happen faster as well.

Whatever you want, if it's growth, more money, or lifestyle success, you've got to get into the game of hiring people and ideally fall in love with it. I believe it's so vital to a business owner that I built my entire mastermind and coaching community around this principle of getting good at hiring great people.

Basically, what I'm saying is that despite the obvious headaches, drama and the unpredictability that comes with hiring people, doing it *right* helps you to live a really great life.

And it can be really fun and rewarding, too.

In my company we talk regularly about the idea of finding "rough diamonds."

This is the entire recruitment strategy that all of my companies are built upon. The exact phrase I use when I talk to my recruitment team is, "Find me another rough diamond."

That's because when we are hiring, we're essentially *mining for diamonds* that simply need a little bit of a polish. We go looking for someone who is capable and already has raw talent, someone who is *already* a star in the making. We look for someone already on the way up who is going to make it somewhere, they just need a few years of being polished in the right environment that promotes success and accountability.

My companies are full of great people that arrived with amazing ambition, great energy, and a strong character that just needed molding.

Or, as I like to say, "sculpting."

@THEPAULGOUGH

I've found a remarkable graphic designer working in McDonald's asking people if they want to "super-size that". I hired an amazing content writer working in a store selling window blinds. The ops manager of my marketing company used to be a teacher and my first-ever employee for my physical therapy clinic I met on the phone when upgrading my mobile phone. True story. I hired a patient with a bad shoulder, who was visiting my physio clinic for treatment, to run my physio business and I've even hired someone who served me coffee every day to run my entire company's hiring and oversee culture.

What I am saying is great people are not always in the place you assume. Like diamonds, if everyone knew where to find them, everyone would be rich. But most aren't and it's because they don't look in the right place.

The secret is to be always looking hard enough and for long enough.

You must prioritize your time to do this right. Every time you go for a coffee, or out to buy some new blinds for your house, drive to McDonald's for a milkshake or call your phone provider, remember that you *could* be talking to someone who *could* help improve the quality of your business, and life.

Basically, as an entrepreneur, you're always looking for the next opportunity to grow your business. It's people who do that for you.

It goes without saying that I've also lost a few of these great people along the way, as their own ambition grows. Some have quit when I least expected or wanted it, and sometimes, they've even gone on to work for a competitor.

And you know what?

So what?

I love that too. Aside from the initial disappointment that I don't get to work with them every day, I take pride in the fact that people come into my world and leave it as stronger, more confident people.

I can honestly say that I've had dozens of people come into my company and leave a few years later much more assured in their life and better at what they do at work. And it's something I am very proud of.

When I get *that email* from an employee expressing their intention to leave, I never react. Detachment is a big trait for any business owner to possess. Besides, I've usually anticipated it. If you pay enough attention, most people have quit before they've actually told you. Their attitude towards being helpful changes, their morning alarm clock stops working, their dog suddenly gets long covid, and they'll start talking trash about others they once liked.

That's just three or four of the things I notice change when someone is about to quit.

Although a little disappointed, and as tempting as it is to think about the negative consequence to the company, I immediately remined myself that I am an amazing *talent spotter* and that the cycle of finding the next diamond in the rough is about to start over again. It's part of the story. All perfectly normal.

If a good employee is leaving, and I'm disappointed, I remind myself that I probably had something to do with *how* they became so good in the first place and that bit isn't leaving the company. I am in some way responsible for their success in the role and I know how to repeat that.

Great football managers build multiple teams with many different players coming and going over the years, but mostly they play the same way. The DNA remains because of the coach.

And likewise, it's the DNA of the company that is responsible for the long-lasting success that goes beyond any single employee. You, the CEO, are responsible for that. Never forget it. It's your ultimate advantage.

How Manage Your Employees to High Levels of Success

If you are going to commit to hiring and managing more people, here's my best advice: Get ready for a *lot of heartache and learn to live with sleepless nights*.

No, I'm only joking…

Here it is, really: The trick to managing employees is to stop seeing them as employees and start seeing them for what they really are—people.

It's important to understand the difference between the two. Here's how I see it:

Employees do tasks required of the business and they get paid at the end of the month for doing so.

People have lots of emotions and typically spend all day long working out *how they feel* about the circumstances of their lives (as well as what role their boss and the company they work for are playing in all of that.)

And it's these emotions that often get in the way of people being great employees.

I sincerely believe most people really do want to be successful and do a good job for their bosses. No one ever wakes up aspiring to be incompetent. Not even politicians. The problem for most people is that they can't deal with how they feel about things happening *elsewhere* in their lives as they come up.

Your project might be the most important thing to you and your business—but it will always come a distant second to an issue in a relationship at home.

It's my belief that when all is said and done, what really separates an *unreliable*, *unproductive* employee from a *superstar* on your team is their ability to handle the pressures of life outside of the office. That reveals their character. The stronger it is, the more they can deal with adversity or things happening they wish weren't.

It isn't about what they do when they feel good, it's what they do when they feel low. That's how you really find out how good your employees are.

The difference in employees being good or bad isn't just found in their capability to the job—it's found in their ability to handle everything else going on around them. And, crucially, how they feel about all of that.

They can have all the telephone skills and techniques you could wish for, but if that person is struggling with something in her personal life, you haven't got a chance of them converting new leads like you hope. There's no amount of training you could ever do to make up for the fact that someone on your team just found a statement for a *maxed-out* credit card they didn't even know their husband had taken out.

There's no point asking someone why the latest project is so bad, and then letting them blame something like a "lack of training", when the real reason is they've just split up with their wife and couldn't focus on the project for worrying over if she was going to run off with someone else.

And if you think I am elaborating in any way with either of these two examples—the breakup and the unknown credit card—you either haven't employed anyone or you're probably still listening to and believing an employee who tells you that your systems and processes aren't good enough. Even though you've updated them seven times in the last three years.

Because *that* is nearly always what happens when they are struggling with something at work: they blame your systems and process. It's never going to be anything else. It can't be anything else. If it's something at home, it means they must face up to fixing it.

If it's your systems, *you* have to fix it. If it's your crappy on boarding process, *you* have to sort that.

It's why the trick to managing people is to start seeing people for what they really are: *human*. And all human beings are imperfect. Not in who they are spiritually, or in their own true nature. That is not what I am getting at. People are meant to be exactly as they are right now.

What I mean is that all humans are *fallible*.

Fallible in the way of keeping their emotions in check, being consistent in their performance, and their ability to be dependable 100 percent of the time.

Every one of us has experienced waking up and feeling good one day, and then waking up the next day unable to work out why you don't feel as good as yesterday.

It's on the day you don't feel as good that you get to see that emotional, unpredictable side of being human. How well it's handled often determines how good of an employee you've got. As I have learned over the last few decades of life, we are all *predictably irrational*, *wildly emotional* at times, and although capable of so much, *not as smart* as we think we are.

A true, if not flattering, reflection of who we all are that when accepted allows us to move forward and make progress regardless.

The thing to remember is employees are people who have the same highs and lows in their lives as you do. They have the same drama with family and issues with friends as you (and me!) and they each react differently to it. It means no one is ever really operating at 100 percent of their capability, 100 percent of the time. Not even you, the immortal, infallible, super-human business owner that you believe yourself to be.

It's certainty true for me.

I'm definitely not capable of firing on all cylinders every single day.

However, it *is* fair to say that I probably am capable of something like 90 percent, 90 percent of the time. And that's the simple standard I shoot for. If I can be at 90 percent of my best, 90 percent of the time, over a twelve-month period, I'll probably have a really productive year.

Accepting this meant I had to adjust my expectations for the people on my team.

Rather than *expecting* and *demanding* 100 percent from everyone, these days I have a very simple philosophy: If I can get 80 percent of their best work, 80 percent of the time, over a twelve-month period, I know I'm going to do very, very, well in my business that year. I am baking into the calendar year the inevitable losses of productivity that will come thanks to the issues people on my team will face in their lives.

It doesn't mean I accept poor standards. No. It means I look at the individual across a period of time and ask how they're performing over months, rather than at an isolated incident or a bad day.

It's a bit like judging a marketing campaign. If you look at Google Ads in one isolated month, it might be easy to say it doesn't work. But I bet if you look at it over twelve months, it will be almost impossible to say it didn't work for you. It's the same with good people.

Again, it's about changing the way you see it and, with it, your expectation.

If you do, you'll have a much better relationship with your team, and yourself for that matter, and it'll be much easier to motivate them to do great work for you over the long term, despite the mistakes they make or the "bad days" they have. They'll also be more likely to stay with you for longer and they'll give you more than they would anyone else.

The important thing is to *detach* yourself from whatever it is they say is going on, or wrong, at work and remember that most of your employees' issues are not found at work, they're being *brought* to work.

I've managed more than 100 people in five different businesses in two different countries and all of my *worst* employees have had one thing in common: *unsettled* home lives.

However, my best and most consistent employees also have one thing in common: a *settled* home life. Or, they possess an incredible, almost superhuman ability to accept that their home life isn't great and come to work and get it done regardless. But the latter are *very* rare. I think I've had two maybe three in all my time.

This is such an important point for you to grasp. Especially if you have managers or are looking to hire or develop a manager for your business.

The thing I'm sharing with you, that I want to make sure you understand, is that the best managers of my businesses or divisions are the people who are able to manage their own emotions. They are the ones who don't need me to help them feel better about themselves. All I ever need to do is talk to them about how to get better at managing others, and making each one more productive. Which is their real job.

But it makes sense, right?

If you can't manage your *own* life, how can you manage someone else's?

And yet, this is often overlooked by many business owners who employee managers or directors who haven't yet mastered their own ability to handle their own emotions.

I believe this is why there is so much drama in most workplaces.

Most businesses have managers in place who got the job because they had been there the longest, had a superior technical skill, or because they're very good at managing processes and procedures.

The latter might be admirable and a good skill to have. But managing *people* is very different from managing processes. After all, processes don't talk back or get defensive during a review. Processes don't get divorced, they don't have sick kids, they don't fall out with the process they sit next to over who should go on lunch first, and processes don't ask for a pay raise for "working hard this last year," either.

Which, by the way, never ceases to astound me.

How do people seriously expect a pay raise because they "worked hard?" It's as if they think they'd still be in the job if they didn't.

Anyway, most businesses really don't need their processes to be managed full time. But their people, do. Your biggest expense can walk and talk. Remember that the fastest way to sink a business is to employ too many people who are unproductive. It's why the real job of a manager is to ensure people are more productive—not constantly fix the new onboarding process or looking for new software to manage billing.

The latter (and former) by the way, being one of life's great "tricks" poor-performing employees love to play on inexperienced managers to cover up incompetence.

As we come to a close of the chapter, the lesson here for you is twofold:

If you are struggling with managing your own emotions, now you know why your business is full of high drama and high maintenance.

It's because you are (ouch!).

And, equally, if you *can* manage your emotions, but the people you *hired* to manage others for you can't, well, it's no wonder you've got more politics going on in your office than what's happening in the White House. I'm dead serious when I say your business will *never* grow if you have people in management positions whose emotions need managing.

Your job is not to manage how they feel. It's to coach them on how to get better at managing employees on how to get better at their jobs.

If you're always hearing about drama, constantly "walking someone off a ledge" or having to deal with emotional outbursts from your managers, take it as a given you've got the wrong people in place and they are holding you back. Toss them overboard ASAP.

The following rule should help you decide *when* to push: when all you hear about is drama, the job is too big for the person in charge. However, if all you hear about are *opportunities*, it's very possible the person is too big for the role and should be considered for promotion.

All of this highlights the importance of you working on yourself and understanding yourself—if you want to be a good leader.

Ultimately, the less irrational and more predictable you are with your emptions, the more consistent and detached you are from stupid but anticipated things, the better you will become at managing your people and the more you will thrive doing it.

People also want to work for these types of people. People who have their own houses in order are rare and others want to flock to them. They want to get behind the security that this type of person offers in the hope of getting a bit of that in their own lives. They think that by getting closer to you for long enough, some of your star quality will rub off on them.

And guess what? It often does.

In the end, as always, all roads lead back to you and how you behave. The fish stinks from the head down, as they say. It's why whenever I am asked for a great book on managing other people, I always suggest starting with one on *how to manage yourself*.

It's because the best book for managing people is one that explains how to understand and manage yourself. You have to learn about and fix your own insecurities before you can do the same for anyone else.

It's been my experience that anyone who has done that usually goes on to become a great manager and enjoys the process more than they ever could have imagined.

@THEPAULGOUGH

I have no doubt you can too.

Major Principle of Chapter 9: You can't achieve anything extraordinary on your own. People give you the leverage you need to in life and at work.

For more tips on hiring and recruitment, be sure to read my best-selling book: ***The Hiring Solution: How To recruit Hire and Train World Class People You Can Trust***. Get it direct from me at www.paulgoughbooks.com or find it on Amazon.

ACHIEVEMENT
CHAPTER 10

The Hard Thing About Big Decisions

If you want to know why your life looks the way it does *today*, then look no farther than the decisions you made in the *past*. And if you want to know what your life will look like in the future, look no farther than the decisions you're making *today*. You are *not* a product of circumstances, more over you are a product of your decisions.

Basically, you can blame a lot of things, but the quality and circumstances of your life are directly related to the decisions *you* make—even the decision you make to *not* make one.

That's why it's safe to say that if you're wanting to *elevate* the quality of your life, *elevate* the amount of money available to you, and even *elevate* the enjoyment in your life so there's more of all those things than you have now, then you also need to elevate the quality of your *decision-making* ability.

@THEPAULGOUGH

Decision making is a skill—not in the way society recognizes the skills of being a doctor, a carpenter, or a basketball player, but there's a *knack to it* that makes life easier if you can master it.

Making decisions can be hard. Doing so comes with risk. That's the hard thing about it. The problem is, a bit like time, decision making is one of those things people take for granted. It's so easy to assume how you currently do something is the *only* way to do it.

After all, no one really sits down and talks you through how it can done be done better. I can't remember getting any education on decision making and by the number of bad decisions people make on a daily basis, it looks like I wasn't the only one.

Sure, the importance of getting it right is often pointed out.

I vividly remember my mother repeatedly telling me to go away and "think about the decision I'd just made"—or to "consider the consequences of it"—but she never really explained *how* to do so. Nor did my teachers. I suspect no one told them how to do it either.

Most entrepreneurs want to feel like they're making progress. And to make progress, it helps to remember that it isn't always about making a big, good decision. No. It's as simple as knowing how to *avoid* making a bad one. Commit to making progress and avoid making bad decisions and you'll probably have a very nice life.

The key is to avoid the stupid stuff that sets you back.

All things being equal, if you could go back and undo the bad decisions you've made in your life, I suspect you'd probably be a whole lot richer instantly. Either with money in the bank or more contentment in your life.

It's why I say that *avoiding* a bad decision is just as important as making a good one. It's also why so it's important to know how to make them.

Mistakes With Decision Making

Before we get to what I believe to be the *biggest decision* any entrepreneur can make, let's look at two of the most common mistakes people make with their decision making.

The first is a failure to recognize the need for a different type of decision-making process based on the size and inevitable complexity of the decision.

A major flaw that leads to bad decisions is first and foremost that you do it *on your own*, in your own head. And that's not an environment conducive to making good decisions.

I don't know about you, but anytime I'm talking to myself, in my own head, I always seem to be able to convince myself that what I'm thinking about is a good idea or great decision. It's not like there's anyone up there to question me, is there? It probably explains why every problem I've ever had one thing in common: they started as good ideas.

There's nothing more gratifying than thinking up your own good ideas.

But just because it's gratifying and feels right in your own head doesn't mean it's a good one in reality. It usually just means it's the first one. You solved the problem of needing to make a decision, but it doesn't guarantee it was the right decision.

The other problem is that you make so many decisions on a daily basis, from which way to go in your car, to what to wear for work and what to eat for dinner, that you can't help but think that the way you make one decision is the way you should make them all.

But that isn't true.

It's one thing to make a quick and easy decision on what to wear or where to eat for dinner. But, it's another thing to make a decision on starting a business or hiring an employee, or what to charge clients in your business. Those things probably need to be run through a different filter. There's a different level of complexity to that type of decision, not to mention risk, so it requires a completely different process than the quick and easy ones with little if any consequence.

That process absolutely should include what I call a "second voice" in the conversation. Basically, this is the process of talking it out with someone who is credible and has prior success or experience in that particular area or subject matter.

Utilizing a second voice from a credible person has been one of the "secrets" to my success. I realized a few years back that it was much easier to be successful if I learn from other people's mistakes than to learn from my own.

It's why I've intentionally sought out people who know more about subjects than I do. It's a simple rule that I use in all areas of my life. If I want to be happier, I look for people who are happier than me and I talk to them about how they did it. If I want to make more money, I look for someone whose tax return is bigger than mine. If I want a better relationship, I look for someone who already has one and discover their secrets.

But that isn't how most people do it.

If they do talk it out, it's usually with a close friend or family member who, although well meaning, is probably at a similar level of thinking about life.

What I mean about that is most people get financial advice from people who are equally as poor. They'll ask for opinions on making money from people with no money. They ask for business advice from people running bad businesses. They ask miserable people how to be happy. And, possibly the worst of all, they ask people with no ambition what they think of their big idea or grand plan. Never forget, the fastest way to kill a big idea is to introduce it to a small mind.

Anyway, it's madness, but this is how it works.

People make decisions based on the "advice" they're given by people who are not at the level of life they aspire to get to. You wouldn't ask a person who failed math for advice on algebra, so why would you ask someone who is absent of fun how to find it?

It's a simple change anyone reading this book can make right now.

People might be nice, might love you, and might have your best interests at heart, but it's time to stop asking them to advise you on things they haven't figured out for themselves.

Instead, seek out people who are doing what you want, not just giving their opinion or telling you what you want to hear.

It can be a mentor or a coach that you pay for and meet with regularly.

It could even be a client or customer of your business who is obviously *high rolling* their way through life. If a client arrives in a helicopter for a thirty-minute appointment, flanked by an entourage who lay the floor with red petals as he walks and shine his shoes as he stands and talks, it might be worth asking that person about the subject *thinking big* and not giving a hoot about what others think.

I suspect there'd be at least *something* to learn if you did.

However, if he's been divorced four times and spends more time in the pub than with his kids, might not be worth asking for advice about raising your family.

Anyway, here's one final point on this: when asking people for advice, from anyone, make sure that the person you're talking to about your next big decision does not rely upon you financially or emotionally.

That rules out your staff, probably your partner, and most likely your close family and friends.

See, anyone who relies upon you to pay their bills, or for the safety and security you bring to them in a relationship, is never going to be able to give you the type of candid, blunt, and direct advice that you probably need to hear for fear of you not liking what they say and therefore losing their emotional or financial lifeline. The type I'm sure you'd get from the guy arriving in the helicopter with the entourage.

When in doubt, always talk to someone independent of either of those two things.

If you're in business, it's for this exact reason you must be part of a peer group or mastermind community so that you can talk things out with people who don't need you to like them or care that they're right.

Mistake Number Two: What's The Consequence?

The second big mistake people make with their decision making is failing to consider the consequences that they could face because of the decisions they make.

Even if you're not going to seek out a second voice in a conversation, at the very least take the time to sit down with a pen in your hand and do some real thinking about the first, second, and third order actions—or consequences—of something you are considering and then ask if you're OK with all of them.

It's important to understand that nearly all that is good, or bad, about your life is found at the second level of action. It's not the first thing that happens after your big decision, it's the one that is a direct result of that.

Let me explain.

Consider a scenario in which you're going to go out with friends and drink lots of alcohol. The decision was to go out with them in the first place. The first thing that happened as a direct result of you going out and following through on that decision was a fun time with friends. So far so good. A fun time is the first order of action of drinking lots of alcohol. However, the second action is that you'll probably have a bad headache the next day if you drink too much.

This means the decision to drink alcohol with friends should be based on the *consequences* of the alcohol and asking whether you can and want to live with that. If you have a clear day on a Sunday, being hung over might be OK.

But if you have a big project to finish at work by Monday, and you need to be in top shape on Sunday, it's probably not a good one. If you can't get it done, or it's shabby, and you get into trouble with the boss or even lose your job, then that was the *real* consequence of the decision you made.

It's the same with something like gambling.

The first decision to gamble probably fills you with a bit of buzz. The anticipation of winning something more than you bet can make you feel good. However, if you bet more than you can afford and you lose, then the second order consequence means you have to explain to your partner and kids why you risk being evicted because you couldn't afford the rent. Which is not good.

As a general rule, the quality of your life is ultimately determined by what happens at the *second action* level of every decision you make.

And the same type of thing happens in business all the time.

The first decision might seem like a good one, but a closer look at what happens next will tell you more.

For example, the decision *not to* hire someone might mean you have a bit more money in the bank that month. However, if the second order action is that you're stressed, tired, burnt out, and risking health complications, then the decision to not hire someone, even though you kept some money in your bank, was a bad one in the end. The money is no good if you're dead. Unless you want a flamboyant and extravagant funeral, that is.

It is the same with things like investing in mastermind groups or coaching.

It's easy to think *I'll just keep the money*, or not go to the event so you can save the time or expense. And sure, it might mean that month you have a bit more money or time on your hands, but if in three months your business is *still* stuck or has problems that could have easily been fixed by going to the mastermind meeting or getting some type of coaching, then how good of a decision was it really? It likely cost you a lot more in the long run. And the best prizes are *always* found in the long run.

In the end, the quality of all your decisions will be measured by what happens *after* you've made them and then asking whether you want the consequences in your life. It sounds so elementary, but spending some time thinking through what is going to happen next is one of the best things you can do if you want to get to the next level—and stay there.

It's hard to enjoy your life and feel good about it if you're always regretting the decisions you've made or, just as likely, made so many bad ones that you become averse to making any more decisions in the future.

When you get to that point, there's very little progress or momentum and that's another source of the real frustration most people live with every day—especially entrepreneurs addicted to progress.

The Big, Bold Decision Framework

I've heard it said that everything you want in life is on the other side of the decision you *don't* want to make today. And when you think about it, there's a lot of truth to that.

If you are stuck, it's because you can't move on and if you can't do that, it's because there's a decision that you're avoiding making.

It usually means you're in your comfort zone hoping that you can get what you want without ever risking how you currently feel. That's the predicament millions of people in the world are in. In a zone of comfort, secretly *un*happy with it, and wanting something else but not prepared to risk the pillow they're on, just in case the new one isn't as good.

With that said, if life does get going *again* at the other side of your comfort zone, it helps to know how to get beyond it, wouldn't you think?

With that in mind, what I'm going to do next is walk you through an exercise I use any time I need to make a *big, bold, decision*—the kind that really impacts the quality of your life for years to come. The kind that gets you out of your comfort zone without feeling like you're taking a massive risk.

It's a framework that helps to make hard decisions a bit easier.

The key to big decision making is to get to the point of making one —and being OK with whatever happens. It's not always about having to get it right—it's about being OK with it going wrong. Sounds a bit strange when you first hear it, but it's true.

See, my definition of a great decision is being in a position after you've made it where you are happy with any outcome. It's when you are comfortable with outcome A, *and* outcome B, that you will have a real quality of life. This is when you're really in control of your life.

The key is to consider what outcome A *and* B (or even C) could be.

We can't always get decisions right—and many times we don't need to. We just need to consider how we would feel if we got it wrong or it doesn't go according to plan. After all, it's not necessarily the actual result of the decision that affects you, it's mostly how you *feel* about it. A common theme throughout this book that comes up too many times to be ignored or dismissed.

The circumstance that follows the decision is one thing, but whether you can live with that is what matters most. What do I mean by this? Well, just think about how many people are right now *still* feeling bad, guilty, or regretting a decision they made months or even years ago.

The circumstances have likely moved on but how they feel hasn't.

That low mood or negative feeling is getting in the way of them feeling good about themselves and that in turn is getting in the way of progress and momentum in their life. It's not the "thing," it's the feeling bad about the thing.

As we covered in an earlier chapter, it's this negative feeling that keeps you stuck. When you go into your head to consider *how you feel about how you feel,* it's really hard to come out. You're stuck in your head trying to work things out and life stands still while you're there.

To get to the point where you are OK with both A and B (even C), the trick is to consider not *only* the good that might come of your decision, or the consequence of it going wrong, but to ask what the *probability* of it is. Then, most important of all, ask yourself **whether or not you can live with that consequence.** It's here that you will know if you should make the decision or not.

Asking yourself and answering honestly whether you can live with a decision going wrong—outcome B—is probably the most important question you'll ever ask.

Those questions form part of a framework that has allowed me to make better and faster decisions—without procrastinating, agonizing, and deliberating for months on end. It means taking the time before making any decision to ask a series of five questions to get to the point where you know if you're OK with something happening that might not be your ideal outcome. Here is the framework for you to look at:

1. "What is the benefit of the decision?" (i.e., "What good could happen if I make this decision?")

2. "What is the probability of that happening?" (i.e., 70%)
3. "What is the negative consequence of this decision?" (i.e., "What could go wrong?")
4. "What is the probability of that happening?" (i.e., 30%)
5. "If it were to come true, can I live with that consequence?"

Now you're familiar with it, let's work through this framework together as we hypothetically hire a new person for your company.

The first thing to ask is: "What is the *benefit* of the decision?"

In the case of hiring, it could mean that customer service is improved and because of that more customers will spend more money. Additionally, staff morale will be boosted because the rest of the team is not stressed out by extra work. It could result in an additional $10,000 per month.

The next question is, "What is the probability of that happening?"

Well, with hiring, you will never get it right 100% of the time. But if you follow the right process and get the right person, the chances of it being a success could be as high as 70%.

The next thing to ask is, "What is the *negative* consequence of this decision?" In the case of hiring, the downside is that they might turn out to be utterly useless, mess a few processes up, lose a few clients, and cause one of the other staff members to quit.

Then, the next question is, "What is the *probability* of that happening?"

It's unlikely *all* of that will happen, but it's possible some of it will.

So let's say it's a 20% chance.

Based on all of this, you can now ask the final question. And here's the most important thing: you must answer it in a heartbeat. Don't think about your answer, simply ask the final question: "If it were to come true, can I live with that consequence?" and within one second, you will know the answer. It's a simple yes or no and you must go with your first answer.

If you work through it and you decide you *can* live with the downside, then you must make the call and do it. Learn to trust your instincts. The best entrepreneurs have amazing instincts. It's just that they don't always take the time to listen to them properly.

The best part of all of this is that because you've considered the downside, there's less chance it will happen. By default, you will have contemplated a few of the risks that could cause it to go wrong and be able to work toward mitigating each one.

And besides, even if it does go wrong, it won't affect you as much as if you hadn't thought it through. That's because if something does go wrong and you didn't expect it to, you spend time asking *why* it went wrong instead of what you need to do to fix it.

Think about this: if you keep asking, "Why did it happen?" it takes you longer to get to the better question that creates instant progress, "What am I going to do now that it *has* happened?"

I challenge you to look at *any* area of your life where asking this question wouldn't be better for you than asking "why." After all, the problem is not the real problem. The problem is you didn't expect or want it.

The Biggest Decision of Your Entrepreneurial Life

Even if you have a decision framework like this, and you actually use it, it still takes a lot of *courage* to make the most important decisions in your life.

Courage is a word that keeps on cropping up in this book.

As an entrepreneur, you need a lot of it to overcome your own insecurities, not to mention the judgment you face from others who question your ambition and don't understand why you live the way you live. There's others, but these three alone can make real progress difficult to come by for any entrepreneur.

Take away the prying eyes of the world and give yourself permission to be OK with failing and I bet your life would be a lot easier to enjoy, would it not?

After all, failure isn't the problem. The issue is how you think others will perceive you if you do fail.

The interesting thing about courage is that it's a lot like character. It absolutely can be developed. The trouble is it can also be easily *lost*. Every time you make the easy, cowardly decision, you weaken your ability to be courageous. And equally, every time you make big, bold, difficult decisions, you develop your ability to be courageous.

This means if you start *avoiding* making hard decisions in favor of easy ones, you may end up losing the ability and never getting it back.

This possibly explains why so many people get to a certain point in their lives and are never able to make the decisions they need to advance.

They literally lost the ability to be courageous in favor of making easy decisions that became their default. Usually done so in favor of seeking *harmony*, *being nice* for the sake of being liked, or keeping *others happy* to avoid conflict. Fine. It's how many like to behave. But you should know that all of these things are the enemy of progress and success.

It's yet another reason why people end up with lives they don't recognize. They are literally living lives made up of lots of little, easy, cowardly decisions instead of lives made up of a few big, bold, and courageous decisions.

If you pushed me, I'd say that courage is the thing you need the most if you're going to really enjoy your life—one you can call your own. It's not money. It's not more time. It's courage. If you've got the courage, the money will make its way to you.

It takes courage to live free from guilt. It takes courage to break social norms and flout outdated rules. It takes courage to live a life that is different from anyone around you. It takes courage to start things that you're not good at and keep going until you are.

It also takes a lot of courage to make a big, bold decision about who you'll hang around with and spend your time with. This is arguably the biggest decision you will ever make in your entrepreneurial life.

That's because if you want to get to the next level of life, you can't exclusively hang out with people who don't want to get there themselves.

They say you're the sum of the five people you hang around with. And I believe it. I made the leap from doing "OK" in life to living a life that 99% of the planet could only dream of simply because I made the decision to change *who* I surrounded myself with on a regular basis. But it wasn't easy. I left the crowd of friends I grew up with and to a certain degree I had to limit even some of the interactions I had with family.

Nature is important. But nurture can't be ignored either. I'd argue it's more important. When it comes to *nurture*, we pick up the most from the people we are around and how they behave or think can easily make its way into our own ways of living. It's why it is important to give some consideration to what you're getting from the people you're close to.

If the people you're surrounded with are living their best lives, have a permanent smile on their faces, can deal with setbacks and adversity like it's a stroll in the park, and they're cashing $50,000 checks for fun, you're in the right group.

Stay there.

However, if the people you're talking to daily are mostly *negative*, *miserable*, and *broke*, it might be worth considering how much their view of the world is rubbing off on you.

Found yourself a little negative or down lately? Ask yourself how many of the people you talk to are the same.

If the people you hang out with have a skeptical, stoic view of life and tell you things like "money does not grow on trees" (even though it does—after all, paper comes from trees), don't be surprised if you adopt that same view.

If the people you hang out with focus more on what they *lack* and believe a good life is something reserved for a "lucky few," don't be surprised if that's how you start to think too.

It's worth considering how most of the people you're surrounded by today actually got there. It was probably *without* any real effort or thought going into it in and I'll go as far as to bet you didn't interview them for a position in your life.

What I mean is we often end up with people based on the school we went to, the area of town in which your parents choose to buy a house, or people already in the office when you started. It's all passive. This means you can end up in social circles that feel comfortable and safe, are nice and friendly, are with people who think at the same level, or earn the same level of income, without much thought or effort going into it.

That's what I mean by there being a *passive nature* to how the people in our lives get there. It's rarely deliberate.

It means unless we're really lucky, and the stars aligned to put you in a group of people who are "smashing it" at life, laughing all the way to the bank, knocking over their life goals for fun, happy at home and with themselves, chances are you might need to do a little "self-selecting" or start the "redundancy process" and change who you should be talking to more often.

To be clear, I'm not saying to cut yourself off from others completely, just to be really careful of how you're allowing yourself to be *influenced* by them.

It might seem nice to stay close to your friends, but if they are mostly negative in how they think about life and what is possible, it means all of your conversations end up being equally negative, often about small, petty problems or idle gossip and not about *big ideas* or *radically* different ways of thinking that could take your life into a different place.

Ideally, the next level.

Interestingly, if you pay attention to the conversations that the people close to you are having, it will reveal a lot about the level of success they're having in their lives. I'd go so far as to say that if I listened to your friend group for sixty minutes in a bar, I bet I could tell what success they're having just by *what* they talk about.

Let's have some fun with this. Below, I'll briefly describe the three different types of people you could spend time with. See how many of your friends and family you recognize as you work through the groups:

Group 1: Unsuccessful People (talk about other people)

If the group of people you're involved with only ever talk about *other people*, take it as given you're in a group of very unsuccessful people. There's nothing interesting going on in their own life and so it's much easier to comment on and pass judgement on others.

They'll be pretty down about most things, and nothing will ever seem to go right for them. They'll be great at the bar, with alcohol in front of them, but at home, in private, expect them to be very "low mood" and mostly skeptical about life.

Group 2: Averagely Successful People (Talk about what they own or plan to buy)

If the group of people you're involved with only ever talk about what they've bought or want to buy, you're probably in a group of *averagely* successful people.

They have a bit of success going on that is usually in the form of a higher-than-average salary, maybe a bigger-than-average house, and it makes them feel good to talk about the things they can buy or have bought.

However, what you find from this group of people is that they live with a lot of resentment and jealousy.

They're doing OK in life when it comes to money and stuff like that, but they struggle *with acceptance of themselves* as they always think they should be doing better than others in terms of what they've got or are able to buy, as that's how they measure their worth.

They live with a lot of "sugar highs" when buying thing or getting things, but are usually not genuinely happy people, or happy for others. It is through gritted teeth that they'll congratulate you on getting your new car. And *oh yeah*, it will be followed very quickly with when they're buying a bigger or better version of it.

Group 3: Successful, Happy, and Fulfilled People (talk about big ideas)

And last but not least, we come to the group you want to be in. You will know you are in a group of *very* successful people when all they ever talk about is their big ideas and the things they're working on to make life and business even better.

They don't really talk about the new car they just bought, they just arrive in it and toss the keys to for the Bentley Continental to the valet guy so they can get on with finding out who's got a big idea they need to know about.

They're not interested in gossip, hearsay, social scandals, or anything like that. All they want to know is what's good, what's working well, and what they could be doing to have more fun in life.

"How Big Is Your TV?"

So, I'm eager to know, did you recognize anyone from reading that? Did you confirm your intuition about your friend's husband, the boring one, who never stops talking about what he wants to buy or telling you how much he makes?

Or, perhaps you spotted your mother (gasp!) in there who does nothing but talk about what others are doing and how they're living their life?

Most of all, I hoped you spotted at least one or two people who only ever want to talk about ideas and big plans? They are the people you need to talk to more.

Anyway, if that didn't help you decide if you're in the right group, another simple and very fun way to determine it is to ask about the size of a person's *TV*. This being a metaphor for the idea that someone who watches more than they read is unlikely to be the person to talk to about important things in life.

If the TV is bigger than that of their *library*, then take it as a given you need to limit conversations with that person to ones of football, scandal, and celebrity gossip.

Don't start talking about money, finding fulfilment, or anything important like that because you won't get much good advice coming back. You'll get opinions, but not much real-world truths you can use. They might tell you what someone like Beyoncé is doing to her lips and teeth, and other good stuff like that, but that'll be about it.

On a serious note, the best group to be part of is the one where big ideas and strategies are shared freely. You want to spend more time with people who don't care too much about buying new things and stuff and have little if any interest in what others are doing or saying.

Which group are you currently spending most of your time with, I wonder?

Before I close out the chapter, let's review what we've covered. The biggest shift in my life happened when I shifted my *thinking* about what was possible for my life. And that happened simply because I changed who I was talking to.

I made the big, bold, courageous decision to spend much of my own money—profits from my physical therapy business—on business coaching, peer-peer mastermind groups, and spending as much of my time as possible with people who were already playing at the level of life I wanted to get to.

This changed my mindset and belief in what was possible for "someone like me."

I had to move from what you might call "realistic" thinking, embedded in me by society and the people around me, and replace it with the more useful "possibility" thinking that I picked up from others living at the level I wanted to live.

It also made it much easier to go and get the life I knew I could live simply because I could see others doing it. Being around them made it easy to do this one simple thing: *ask them how they did it.*

I sometimes wish I could say it was more difficult than that, but it wasn't. Sure, I had to go and do the work. But that was the easy part. Figuring out what to work on is always the hardest part. If you look at most people's lives, they're running east to find a sunset. Which isn't going to happen. A simple way of explaining that they're doing a lot—like that "busy" thing we spoke about earlier in the book—but they're mostly busy working on the wrong things. I think the term "Busy fools" sums it up nicely.

Major Principle of Chapter 10: The quality of your life stands and falls on the decisions you make. The biggest decision you'll make is determining who you will allow to influence you.

PART 3

ACHIEVEMENT
CHAPTER 11

When They Zig, You Zag

I often say that simplest path to success in life is to look around at what everyone else does—and then do the *complete opposite*. If you see a big group of people going one way, it's probably best to go the other. If there's a popular opinion that has been adopted by mainstream media or the masses, take it as a given that the opposite stance is going to be more useful.

After all, if you do what others do, you'll get what others get.

The biggest problem with popular opinions is they are easy conclusions to come to. A bit like rules, there's no thinking required and because thinking takes effort and uses up more oxygen than anything else you can do, people like to skip it whenever they can.

It's also why popular opinions last for decades—even centuries. Even though the *facts*, the *data*, and the *statistics* do not support the assumption or the opinion, somehow these popular opinions seem to live on and be passed on from one generation to the next.

There are a significant number of multi-millionaires in the world who *never* went to college, but apparently the only way to earn a good living or get a good job is if you go to one and get yourself into $100,000 worth of debt.

There is a divorce rate of about 50% in the first three years after marriage, but apparently the only way to be happy these days is to get married.

There's an eight-year-old opening and playing with toys on YouTube every morning who is worth $50,000,000, but apparently there's no opportunity for kids anymore.

On and on the proof goes of people defying popular assumptions, often making a mockery of the popular opinions, but for some reason people choose to overlook the evidence.

And as I say so often say these days, *none of this makes sense to me*.

What people tell me about how life works and what I see with my own eyes are often two very different things. It's why I would encourage you to have faith in the things you can see, not just the things you can't.

Most of the things you need to know about living a good life are staring you in the face every day. They're hiding in plain sight. They're also often the opposite of what *most* people want you to believe.

A System Designed to Keep You Stuck

You don't have to look all that closely to see that the way most people are living doesn't work. Not if *prosperity* and *enjoying life* are the goals. I don't hold back in saying that the system that was designed for you many years before you were born simply isn't working.

We're all told that the system is designed *for* us and that if we all behave like good little boys and girls and follow the rules, then we'll all get our rewards in the end. But it's complete rubbish. And I'll prove it to you in a moment. The system is not working *for* us. It's actually more accurate to say it's happening *to* us.

The system has never worked and never will for this simple reason: **the system is held together by *fear* and *compliance*, which makes prosperity and opportunity almost impossible to achieve.**

Think about this: we're all fed into the same system, with the same accepted ideals and ways of thinking and living, but how many truly *happy*, *fulfilled,* and *independently successful* people is this system producing? I bet that despite knowing hundreds of people, you won't need more than one hand to count them out.

Seriously, ask yourself just how many people you know are really living a terrific life versus simply surviving and barely making it through.

At best, most people in the western world are living just below what you might call the "Revolution Line."

They've got *just* enough to survive, *just* enough to get by, and just enough to justify the struggle. Even though people know they are dissatisfied with what they're getting, they're not dissatisfied *enough* to start a mutiny and overthrow the system, just in case they lose what little they've got. Given the choice, most people prefer certainty over uncertainty. Even if it means *certain* unhappiness.

@THEPAULGOUGH

As a kid I used to play a video game called Lemmings. If you don't know it, look it up on YouTube. The way most people live their lives reminds me of that video game and how the lemmings all behave. Which is basically to follow the lemming in front—wherever it goes—even if that lemming is headed for a ditch or off a steep cliff to a certain death.

All the lemmings are the same size, so the lemming in the back can't see what the one in the front can—the danger.

But each one assumes that because the one in the front is headed a certain way, then it *must* be OK. The lemming behind the one in front thinks that no one is so dumb that they'd walk themselves off a cliff or down into a big ditch and stay stuck there—but the lemmings do. And they keep on doing it no matter how many lemmings die.

If one goes one way, it's not long before everyone else follows. In the end, there are hundreds of them all following the one in front to their eventual death or demise, with not one of them questioning why.

To bring this story out of video game land and into the real world, the same thing is happening in society with real people. One person blindly following the one in front, no matter how silly it is to do so.

In society, people aren't really following each other off a literal cliff to certain physical death. It's more of an *emotional* death. It's a life where emotions are out of control, frustration rules, and days lack real and genuine fulfilment.

And yet, to avoid this, all you really have to do is the complete opposite of what everyone else around you is doing. It's as simple as learning to *"zig when they zag."*

Sure, it's easier said than done, but if there ever is anything you "must" do, it's this.

I've been *zagging* for a very long time and I can assure you it's a lot of fun, a lot more carefree, and I get to live my own life. Which is nice.

Has Anything *Really* Changed?

Despite how easy it is for me to say, *"zig when they zag"*, I appreciate it's also really hard to do so. That system I referred to above is a tough one to escape. From the minute you're born, you are part of it whether you like it or not.

You *will* be entered into an organized way of living that suits the masses, promotes control, and statistically gives you almost no chance of prosperity, whether you like it or not. It's the rule.

This system was created hundreds and hundreds of years ago, probably sometime around the year 1550, and I have no doubt it was a system that was appropriate for the times.

What times?

Well, a time when there was little if any knowledge around about how life and the world *really* worked; a time when people really *did* believe that a storm in the sky meant the world was going to end and even had some people believing the storm was put there to punish the people below for having done some "evil deed."

Even then, way back in the 16th century, there were obviously one or more ingenious souls who cottoned on to the fact that if you want to control someone, then all you must do is promote fear.

According to this amazing system they created, everyone in the village was kept under control by a few people. For the purposes of this rather elaborate account of life back then, let's call them the "Elders."

These Elders were either born into wealth or had the biggest, most powerful families in the village. These Elders also had the most important thing of all: the ability to keep a *straight face* while telling people why inclement weather meant someone in the village must have done something really bad, and this bit of a storm is the big bad weather god extracting revenge.

See, back then, everyone was lacking in a bit of what you might call "real and credible information." I wasn't around in the 16th century, but I'm going to go out on a limb and suggest that there was probably a *genuine* limit to the understanding of how life really worked, how weather systems were created, and how to live life to the fullest.

To cut them all a bit of slack, they probably didn't even know that those things in their heads were brains, never mind how to use them. All they knew was if something looked like a lion it was going to kill them and if it looked like a cow they could kill *it* and eat it. Now that does make sense to me.

Anyway, this *naivete* of the villagers played right into the hands of the Elders, who were much smarter than the rest. They knew the rain and thunder seemed to happen whenever it got a bit hot and sticky, and that it didn't really mean a load of people needed to die. But they kept it to themselves regardless and used the occasional area of *low pressure* to ensure people complied.

It meant the system *they* created, to suit *them*, was left alone, mostly unchallenged.

After all, no one would dare. Not if the threat of certain death from a bit of light drizzle was hanging over their heads.

It also meant there wasn't all that much of a revolt, there were no uprisings or any protests—they didn't even have pens or crayons to write "*Elders Out*" or "*We Want Change*" on placards. Even if they could write, they wouldn't do it out of fear of another bit of rain pounding down on the village and killing everyone.

This meant the Elders and the two or three other wealthy families in the village were free to tell everyone how to live, and they knew they could get away with it.

It meant society became a bit more organized, and humans continued to live on for a few more centuries. Villages became towns with nice-looking squares for the Elders to stand in and preach their stories of fear and compliance. Everyone bought into the idea that "good" human beings all *did as they were told* and eventually towns became cities with lots of people living in them, all doing as they were told.

Soon there were banks and schools, and people got these things called jobs and everyone was told they were part of something that the Elders called "progress."

Progress became such a big thing in society that Walt even created a carousel ride in honor of it at Disney World.

You get to sit in it for twenty minutes and if you don't get dizzy as you loop around, you learn about how far we've all come in the last couple hundred years. It really is magical. Ironically, the ride starts with a power cut caused by some bad weather, but nobody worries about dying—only if they're going to be able to watch TV.

See, I told you we'd made progress.

If you haven't been on it yet, I recommend you ride it quickly as they'll no doubt take it out soon. Someone will likely be offended by the very idea of what appears to be a perfectly happy family making progress.

Anyway, so far so good.

Except here we are in the 21st century with the same type of thing still happening.

A system that organizes billions of people into a way of living that suits a *small minority* of people, organized around fear and compliance, everyone duped into thinking that they've got a say in any of it. The small minority now being the governments, corrupt politicians, the banks, and a few hundred families who control most of the wealth on the planet.

And you can now add to that list the owners of the social media apps who want to tell everyone how to think—and even how to vote.

But what about everyone else, I hear you cry? What happens to the other seven billion or so people on the planet? How are they supposed to live?

Well, they are all told to be grateful for what they get or risk being labeled as greedy or selfish if they want anything more. And if they do get more, they'll have to give at least half back in taxes. More if you live in New York or California.

Everyone else is given small handouts to make survival possible. Everyone else is made to feel guilty for everything they say or do, forced to live a life where they regret every decision they ever make, or don't make, and told to fear the future as "the good old days" are in the past.

And *oh yes,* they are also told that they are incapable of surviving outside of the pack, forcing them to stay inside it, ensuring the system lives on.

@THEPAULGOUGH

Aaaaah, the sweet smell of centuries of progress!

Now look, I know what you're thinking.

It's either, "Does Paul own a time machine like Doc Brown from *Back To The Future* and did he go back in time to see how it all worked in the 16th century?" or, "It sounds like nothing much has really changed since the 16th century."

And if it's the latter—that not much has really changed in all these centuries—then you'd be right. Not much really has changed between the 16th century and the 21st century.

And that's the point I am trying to make.

In a rather comical but *somewhat* serious, far-fetched but *somewhat* true kind of way, I'm pointing out that *fundamentally*, nothing much has changed.

The 21st century version of the Elder, with the ability to keep a straight face about the likelihood of someone needing to die if the weather is bad, is a politician telling you that the world will end if big government doesn't pass a law to stop it.

It's the founder of a social media app influencing how people think to suit his agenda for control.

It's also a news editor who decided three weeks ago how she wants you to think *today*, to suit her agenda for "humanity."

An example? If the editor in my state decided covid *wasn't* a risk, people in my state went outdoors. If the editor in the neighbouring state decided she though it *was*, millions of people never left the house *or*, let anyone in.

I heard it got so bad in some states that *Santa Claus* himself wasn't even allowed in homes unless he'd had a negative test 24 hours before, and all his reindeer wore masks.

Poor Rudolf was banned from all states though—except Florida, of course—even if he was negative and had all *six* boosters. His *bright red nose* was on the list of symptoms that meant he needed to "shelter at home" in Lapland. Despite having had that same red nose for hundreds of years, no official cared. Just in case.

Of course, I am exaggerating, a *little*, but I'm not too far off with some of the madness that goes on in this world today.

Anyway, back to it, it's also a banking system that, from the minute you are born, wants you to have your own account and a credit card with a pre-approved limit on it so that you can get into debt early, and then spend your whole life begging for a bit more from another bank to pay that bank back.

It's an education system that promotes memorizing facts and obedience instead of critical thinking and how to sell, communicate, prioritize, or manage emotions. And that's before I get started on the "agenda" that some governors think schools are better suited to teach than a kid's own parents.

It's a college system that wants all parents to "proudly" wear its apparel, just to make sure the kid doesn't drop out. Little Jonny might be thinking about it, but he won't leave and get that job he *really* wants if it means his mom can't wear that t-shirt anymore.

And by the way, if you think I'm being cynical here, I regard this type of thing to be one of the greatest marketing ideas I've ever seen.

"How do we increase stick rates at our very *expensive* college?"

"I know, let's make this about the kid disappointing his parents if he tries to leave. That *pressure* should do the trick!"

I could go on and on. These people and how they dictate to society haven't changed—they're just holding new titles.

Like it or not, in one way or another, we're still organized around fear and control and we're still living in a world that requires compliance with rules created by Elders none of us have ever met.

And *yet*, so much *has* changed.

So much *has* improved and so much *has* happened to mean that people don't have to feel shackled to this broken system.

For starters, we now know that an area of *low pressure* means just that—it's an area of low pressure—and it's nothing that anyone has done or not done. Best, they can even predict it coming a few weeks ahead of time to give everyone notice to get inside and avoid getting wet.

There are now these things called books and libraries with information in them about how life works and how to make lots of money. You can even get them delivered to your house with the click of a button on your phone.

There's this thing called the internet that makes accessing information or talking to other people happen in less than a second. There are reliable teachers of real-world information, with real-world experience, willing to share profound truths and they're easy to find and reach with one search on Google—available on a free computer in a free library.

It isn't about getting "a" job (singular) anymore.

There's the ability to get multiple jobs, to bring in multiple streams of income, while you sleep, to ensure that debt is kept only to the type of *good debt* you might use to buy a home. And it's never been easier to find those jobs either. You can apply while you're in the restroom of a bar waiting for your beer to be served if you don't like the job you've got or want a second. As a bonus, half the world don't want a job anymore so it's never been easier to get a better one.

What I am saying is this: there's more opportunity, knowledge, and access to credible knowledge than ever before. And yet, life is *still* organized into a "one size fits all," hundreds-of-years-old system where very few people make it out or really prosper.

After all, the 1 percent is *still* the 1 percent, isn't it?

Have you ever wondered why, despite all this advancement in technology and things like AI, the internet, an ability to get a job in one country while living in another, a global customer base to market and sell to, or being able to access anything you need to improve your own life or business, 24/7, it's never been the 2 percent?

I say it again, that *doesn't make sense to me.*

But I'll tell you why it happens. And it's simple: it's because everyone is following each other's way of living, hopelessly hoping that the one before is going the right way. A bit like those lemmings I mentioned earlier.

Each one lacking the courage—possibly *permission* —to defy the system and live in their own unique way. An opportunity that in the 21st century is available to us all. You included. No excuses.

The Wealth Pyramid

So just how broken is the system? Just how utterly *useless* is it at helping people live the type of life they dream of and become independently wealthy, able to act freely and live comfortably with the ability to do things and go places that make life more fun and enjoyable, free from ever worrying about the next credit card bill or a mortgage interest rate rise?

Well, it's about as broken as the trust people have in politicians.

Here, let me explain just how bad it is: at the time of writing, the median household income in the U.S. was just under $65,000. The average median net worth of someone 45-55 years old is $125,000. For someone 55-64, it is $187,000.

Forty-four percent of the population pays zero income tax and the top 4 percent of income earners make $309,348. The top 1 percent of income earners make $737,000 and the top 0.1 percent of income earners make just shy of $3,000,000.

I bet most people reading this book would be very happy with a salary of $300,000. And yet, 96 percent of the population do not make that and never will—even if they go to that amazing college and rack up just as much in debt.

This means if you copy what 96 percent of the population do, and how they think, you are unlikely to ever make that type of money. It means if you think and act like the 96 percent—the masses—you will be very unlikely to make this level of money and it means you will probably never get to the point of being independently wealthy. Not unless you inherit it or win the lottery. And I wouldn't like to think I was living my life waiting for either.

This data doesn't read well.

But it gets worse. There's this thing called the *Wealth Pyramid* that gives you a better understanding how bad the system is.

The Wealth Pyramid is a statistical representation—a comparison—of how much cash people have organized into five different levels. One glance at it highlights everything I've just been saying and exposes how nearly *impossible* it is to achieve the type of life you probably really want by following the crowd and staying inside the system.

@THEPAULGOUGH

Here is the Wealth Pyramid. Take a look at it, then I'll explain it to you in a way that makes sense to your life:

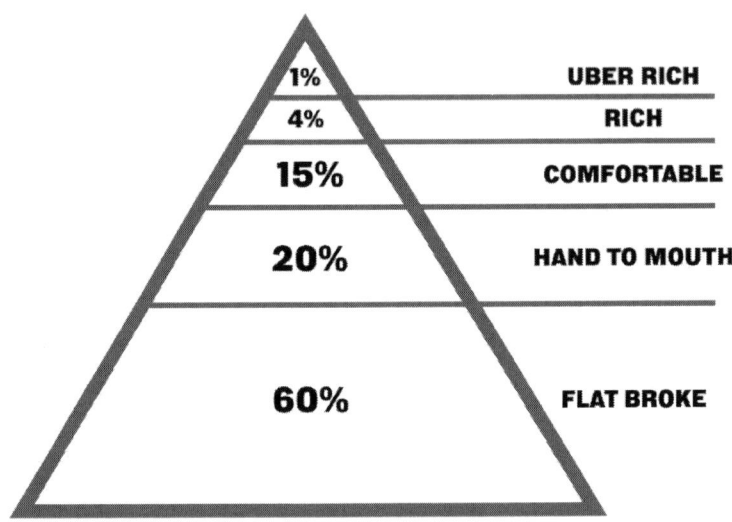

Here's how the Wealth Pyramid works.

Level 1: Flat broke

At the bottom of the pyramid, you find 60 percent of people and they are all broke. They have nothing to fall back on. They don't have a shilling to their name and are relying heavily on hand-outs from the state and possibly even food banks from time to time.

Level 2: Hand to mouth

Next up in the pyramid, sitting on top of those 60 percent, are the 20 percent of people who have only what they make. They live month to month and often they run out of money before the month is up. Or, you could say, there's *more month than money available.*

Level 3: Comfortable with a little left over

On top of those people sit the 15 percent of the population who have some level of savings. They're dependent upon themselves for most things in life. They're not broke and they're not living month to month. They're able to go on a holiday and buy some nice things from time to time. They're not rich, but they are comfortable. They *couldn't* retire on what they've got but they could survive a few months if there was a big storm in their life.

Level 4: Rich and lots of excess

Next up is the 4 percent of the population who are very rich. They could retire right now if they wanted to. They probably have more than one home and they fly first class anywhere they go. They don't need to go to work—they choose to. They could retire but they don't want to because of the thrill they get from whatever it is they do. The feeling they get is more important than the money they make now.

Level 5: Uber rich and anything is possible!

Finally, at the top of the pyramid are the 1 percent. Or the "evil 1 percent" as some in the media like to refer to them. These people are insanely rich. "Filthy rich," as society might say (as if it's somehow dirty to be that rich?). These folks have hundreds of millions of dollars, they have their own planes and a team of people looking after their affairs.

They work—but only from their yachts in the south of France. They're rich beyond anyone's wildest dreams. It's A list movie stars, business tycoons, and top sports stars. They're living the dream and then some.

Why No Change?

Now the wealth pyramid is interesting in and of itself. But the bit that need examining is *why* these levels *haven't changed* in the last fifty years.

Think about how much technology has improved the way we work in the last few decades. We've had the arrival of the internet, where eight-year-olds can become millionaires or business owners can have an almost unlimited customer base.

Think of all the different governments in that time. We've had multiple different presidents or prime ministers; it's changed from red to blue run governments a dozen times over and yet none of them have been able to do much to change any of this.

It's why I have no hesitation in saying that today's governments and politics in general are part of the problem and not the solution. Proving who is right or wrong has become a distraction from making any real difference. It's not about a common goal, it's whose goal is the best goal. Screw agreeing on *how to get to the goal*, it's about fighting over whose goal is the most self-serving and appearing the most noble in the eyes of the public.

And sadly, if there *is* going to be any change, it will more likely be the amount of people at the bottom of the pyramid. It seems more and more people are needing the support of the government, and doesn't the government just love that?

Government believes that what they do is about promoting independence for their people but really, everything they do these days is about creating *dependence* on the government. The more they give people, the more they reduce their ability to help themselves, and in turn, the more people feel compelled to hang on their every word thinking they "need" to.

Government was once about creating a civil, safe, and fair society, and ensuring its citizens were protected from genuine harm—terrorists, pandemics, and the like.

These days it's about freebies and handouts that have become more attractive than most people earn by working. It's now about ruling *over* the country, looking *down* on the people, *telling* people how to think, and dictating what is and what isn't socially acceptable, so much so that people feel they can't do anything *but* depend and rely upon them for everything.

Including when to wear a cloth on your face, who to stand next to, and for how long. Not to mention if you can let Santa into your home and what test he needs to take to make sure "you stay safe this Christmas."

It wouldn't be so bad if any of the people making the rules had lives or intentions that even *somewhat* looked like the intentions and lives of the people they're lording over. When their only intention is power and control, and the people they "serve" want freedom and prosperity, it isn't going to end well. There's a huge disconnect and that frustration you see in society and playing out all over social media is the evidence.

But let me give the politicians at least a bit of credit.

I realize I have spent a good bit of this book bashing politicians, and I wouldn't want you thinking I that I don't see anything good that they do.

That's why I'd like to highlight the thing I think they're really good at. And that is thinking up *ingenious* ways to tax the rich—the ones who made it outside of the system—to fund all this madness. They're amazing at that. Best in the world, in fact.

Anyway, if you want to make real change in your life, you're going to have to do it for *yourself*. You do that by making the decision to live your own life, on your terms, and committing to doing great things for yourself that, when you've done, put you in a strong and powerful position to help others.

As I've said many times before, the best thing you can do for miserable people is decide to not be one of them. Show them a better way. And it's the same with the system. The best thing you can do for the people stuck in the system is decide not to be one of them. Unclog it. Opt out of it. Reduce the lines inside it.

Show people a better way with how you live your own life and how good you feel about it. Never feel guilty about it, either.

And then, when they show up and ask how you did it, be sure to *bill them* for it!

Don't give any of it away free. You'd be *devaluing* the progress you've made and setting people up for failure by letting them think that everything is just going to come their way, freely and easily, without any effort or commitment required on their part.

You know, a bit like how some of the people running the government believe life should be for everyone already.

Anyhow, let's move on to the next chapter and talk about something else that eludes most entrepreneurs—the almighty rainbow titled "work life balance."

Major Principle of Chapter 11: Conventional thinking about life, success, and making money clearly doesn't work. If you're stuck for ideas, or not sure what to do, look at what the majority do and do the exact opposite. The majority are nearly always wrong.

ACHIEVEMENT
CHAPTER 12

Balance Is Bullshit

The idea that you can ever get a "work/life balance" is, quite frankly, complete BS. It's a bit like trying to reach the end of a rainbow—you know it's there somewhere but no matter where you look, you can never seem to find it.

Work/life balance is an *ideal* that is right up there with trying to manage time or thinking you can be happy all the time. Although both sound fantastic in theory, they aren't practical or possible.

Basically, the work/life balance mantra is another one of those popularist ideas that we just spoke about in the last chapter that does nothing but leave people perpetually frustrated in their pursuit of trying to achieve something that never existed in the first place.

The truth is that balance is *bullshit*.

And yes, you absolutely can tell that to your wife, husband, partner, mother, father, and anyone else whose judgemental eyes are fixed permanently on you, questioning how you spend every weekend or how many times you made it back on time for dinner this week.

But I won't just tell you it's OK to do so, I'll even go as far as to explain exactly what to say. I would like to propose something along the lines of the following:

"Honey, I love you, and I appreciate your concern for the *balance* in my life, but look, I've not fallen over in years. Not since I had too many Vodka Mules at your mother's 80th birthday party and you stopped me from ever drinking again."

Seriously, this thing called *balance* might be important to your partner, to your employees, or to a prima ballerina. And sure, it might come in handy if you're ever pulled over by the cops at night and they suspect you've had a bit too much to drink. It might help you avoid going to jail. However, it's not at the top of the list of requirements for an entrepreneur with a desire to grow and succeed.

And the sooner you face up to that, the better.

See, the thing that entrepreneurs want to feel, just as much as a bulging wallet and a pat on the bank from the bank manager, is like they're at least making some progress towards their goals.

It's what we love the most: that amazing feeling you get from growing personally and professionally, coming home at night feeling energized and like you're getting closer to your goals. The problem is that progress is often messy and chaotic. It doesn't like routine. It doesn't like rigidity, it doesn't always have things happening at the same time every day, and it doesn't always go according to plan.

It doesn't come with an alarm clock that tells you when to go home and it definitely doesn't always materialize when you hope it will. It doesn't stop just because the civil servants' clock stopped, and it doesn't care that your kids have a soccer game on a weekend.

Progress has its own rules and they're often opposite to the quiet, simple, and routine life that most *normal* folk prefer.

And by *normal*, I mean normal people, with normal jobs, doing normal things.

Not *weirdos* like you and me who detest routine and normality and prefer the unpredictability, excitement, and heartbreak that comes with business ownership.

If nothing else, remember this: progress is the *prequel* to success.

Progress is made when no one is looking, it's the work you do in private, mostly unnoticed. Success is the thing that they see. It's the car they ride in with you or the big house they visit to watch the game.

Here's the important bit to understand: how success in business and life are *really* achieved is very *different* from how most people were taught.

See, most people learned how to do things in life based on what they were taught in school. Which was mostly to think and act "sequentially." That is where one thing happens, then it is completed, and then something else comes along after.

Think about lessons in school. You finished one, then walked to the next. You finished one school year, then graduated to the next. In the sequential world, you start one thing, give it all your attention, complete it, and then move on the next thing when you're done.

"Do this, *then* do that" is a great way for *some* people to get things done—especially if you are an employee. The thing is, it's *not* so good if you are the owner of the company. You'd simply never get enough things done to get ahead fast enough. As a result, there'd be little if any progress.

That's why the owner of a business needs to learn to live and be comfortable with working on multiple tasks, spinning many plates, fighting many fires, all at the same time. Progress only happens in the entrepreneur's world by learning to do things *simultaneously*.

Basically, you're taking the history lesson at the same time as the English, math, science, and geography lessons.

Is it messy? Of course it is.

And that's the fun of it—learning to deal with it all and, equally, learning about yourself as you figure out how you're doing.

Sure, you need a bit of structure in your day, like I mentioned earlier in the book, but it also can't be *so* structured that it borders on a military operation. That isn't what entrepreneurs need or want.

I guess what I am saying is that it's all about **recognizing that entrepreneurs need to live one way, and employees another.**

It takes a very different type of person to live simultaneously rather than sequentially, and problems seem to really come to the surface when you partner with, or marry, someone who is an employee and doesn't understand the difference in what is required by both roles. If you're not on the same page, or just don't know the page exists, then it's going to hinder your ability to be as successful as you would like. In both your career *and* your relationship.

It's hard to get creative about your next big marketing campaign when all of your creativity is being used on having to think up different reasons to justify why you're at work, is it not?

The reality of being a business owner—an entrepreneur—is that your life will never be balanced. It's better to accept that and be OK with it starting today.

My view of it is as simple as this: if you're always at work, 24/7, and have been for years, always missing out on important things in your family's life, that's a sign something is wrong. And you don't have a problem with "work/life balance." You have a much bigger problem than that. It's either an *addiction* to being at work, a problem you're not facing up to in your personal or home life (the likes of which we discussed in Chapter 4, "What Drives You On Can Also Drive You Mad") or you don't have a life and probably need to get one.

Each one easy to hide behind, but none are desirable and none are conducive of a life that you could call extraordinary.

The trick is to start to think of yourself a bit like a prima ballerina.

When she stands on one toe, the foot, although you can't see it, is always twitching. It's always moving. She might look perfectly still, but she's not. The muscles and ligaments are always contracting and relaxing to ensure she looks still, but the only way she maintains her balance is if she constantly counterbalances.

That contracting and relaxing is what you and I must do each day, each week, each month, only with our *thoughts* and *time*.

Don't look for the perfect routine—it doesn't exist. Most people who have one are usually mind-numbingly bored and so sick of their lives that they end up doing *silly* things to find excitement. They have achieved the perfect routine, but at the expense of their personalities and zest for life. That went out the window in favor of knowing what every minute of every day needs to look like and forgetting that life is about having fun and not being held hostage to a clock.

If you ask me, the only perfect routine is one that includes constantly looking at your life, considering if it's what you're doing is allowing you to make progress and just as important, how it's affecting the people you love—and *then* doing something about it using the answers you come up with (i.e., make a change to your work week).

Do that regularly, say once per month, and you'll probably find you're going to do just fine at keeping the people around you happy at the same time as making progress towards your goals.

Expand The Box

Personally, I've never *struggled* with work/life balance all that much. That doesn't mean I am not out of sync now and then. I am, regularly. Just ask Natalie if you ever bump into her. It just means I've never *struggled* with it.

Remember, the only difference between effort and struggle is a negative emotion. In this case, that negative emotion is the feeling of guilt.

It's why they never find a fix to the work/life balance thing despite the thousands of books being written on it. They try to fix a feeling of guilt by organizing their calendar, buying an app, conforming to another silly rule, or giving up on essential things every entrepreneur needs—room to breathe, think, and time to get things *wrong*.

Like we discussed earlier in the book: guilt *can* be *great*.

If you use it correctly, that is.

Rather than letting it get to me and making me feel bad, I use any guilty feeling I have about being away with the kids and out of the office—or in the office and away from the kids —as a reminder to question how I am spending my time. I notice how I feel and then simply ask what it means.

The feeling I get forces me to question if what I am doing is the best use of my time and, in that respect, I am making a decision that is right for *today*, for *now*, based upon everything I know to be true about my life and the people in it, *at that time*.

In that respect, I would say that I am *counterbalancing* more than I am balancing.

I accept that I am always falling over, but simultaneously always hoping that I catch myself just in time before I hit the floor. And by falling over, I mean getting out of sync with where I spend my time for too long or so long that it really affects someone, or something, more than it needed to.

What do I mean by that?

Well, let's say I go on holiday for eight weeks with my kids and check out of work completely. I suspect the kids are going to be very happy they got Daddy in the water park or a soccer field for two whole months. However, there might be a big problem back in the office if I check out for that long that I might not want to face when I get back.

And equally, if I *never* come home at night, and am *never* around on a weekend for eight weeks straight, there's probably going to be a bit of a regret there too.

I'm probably going to miss something very big in my kids' lives—even if it's just to be with them for a story before bed and ask how their day was.

Which, as I see it, is a very big deal.

The trick to all this is to *expand the box* you're playing in. Do not put yourself in a rigid box with solid walls and try to live within it. That's what most people do as they want to feel certain about everything. They need to know how everything is going to be, all of the time. They're not in control like that, though. They're abdicating control to a life full of rules and constraints determined in advance.

Take control of your life and build your own box—a metaphor for your own rules and conditions—that allows movement so you can push and *expand* the box that you play in, as and when you need.

Don't try to control yourself to the point that there's no ability to twist or tilt. Instead, I recommend you try to "contain" yourself.

There's a difference between "control" and "contain." Control is dull and boring. And when it's self-imposed, it's madness. Containment is different. It allows for some wiggle room on things and a bit more room to play.

I agree that it's highly possible that if you spend your whole life controlling yourself, being 100 percent disciplined, never being late, always starting and stopping something when you agreed to it years before, then you might make a *bit* more money. And there's going to be someone who makes a lot more money than me saying they did so by living that way.

And that's fine. But remember that it's not just about copying success.

It's about mastering *fulfilment*. Big difference.

Some people with lots of money got there with amazing sacrifice, rigid routines, and never seeing their kids grow up. Good for them. But that's not what I want for my life. I'd rather earn a bit less, but have more fun, more enjoyment, and see my kids play soccer at least once or twice per week. And oh yeah, be OK with being late as time-to-time stuff *does* come up.

Remember, this book—and, life as it happens—is not just about making money. It's about **enjoying it and feeling good about it** as you do.

Personally, I think you need a bit of flexibility and unpredictability to do that.

You need just enough certainty mixed with a dash of *uncertainty* if you want to feel good about life and enjoy it. Too much of one or the other is not good for anyone.

Too much certainty makes you dull and boring, and equally, too much *un*certainty and you'd be a nightmare to live with and probably never get much done. You'd be jumping out of a plane, which is fine so long as you have a parachute on your back, instead of committing to the marketing plan that the business needs to meet payroll.

Don't get me wrong, there must be *some* structure and routine, but if there's too much of it you might as well be working for the government. It's why I am baffled by any entrepreneur who arrives at and leaves work at the same time every day.

Isn't that the definition of an employee? Just a thought.

Anyway, instead of being so rigid, I propose you give yourself a little wiggle room to live as you please with 10 percent flexibility on everything. Maybe even 20 percent.

As I always say to Natalie, "Five o'clock doesn't really mean five o'clock." It means I am *aiming* for five o'clock. She's been with me long enough to *not* expect that I'll be home at the exact time I say I will.

After reading that, I bet your immediate assumption is that I always come home *late*.

Well, sometimes I do, but there are equally days where I come home early. When I need to stay, I stay. When I need to leave, I leave.

I have real control over my days, my life, and my time, and I do it by approaching each day, each situation, and asking, "What do I need to do right now for the greater good of everything and everyone?"

The fact that I'm never home at the same time each day is the best proof that I have control over my day. Deciding today to be home at 6 PM every night next year doesn't work for me. It's too much pressure on my shoulders and doesn't factor in all of the things I don't even know are going to happen yet.

I make the best attempt I can to be with Natalie and my boys when appropriate and I use my own judgment—my ability to think for myself—as to whether or not I need to stay at work that day or that night, work that weekend or not, or if I absolutely *do* have to be home at 5 PM for something I don't want to miss. Like soccer, or just to mess around in the pool if that's what I think is needed.

Expanding the box I play in is one of the best things I've ever done.

I use the principle in all areas of my life and it really makes a difference in its quality. For example, I don't try to be a certain weight all the time. I try to stay within a box that can be expanded from time to time depending upon the circumstances. Sometimes I am 203 pounds, sometimes I'm 207 pounds.

Does it matter *that* much? So much that I should stop living my life or stop eating drinking things that in moderation are absolutely fine?

If I'm going on holiday, or it's the festive season, then I might eat and drink a bit more than normal. As a result, a few extra pounds might be added. But really, who cares? It's nothing in the grand scheme of things of things as the nights out with friends and family are more important to me.

Playing within a box allows me the ability to say, from time to time, "To hell with it tonight, let's do it." Best of all, I'm doing it guilt free.

As I said before, I don't want my life to be a military operation, nor do I want to wake up feeling guilty after doing something I really enjoyed. My life is to be enjoyed, not lived by stupid, self-imposed rules. Playing within a box that *I* built, that can be expanded from time to time, helps me do that.

However, here's the thing: if three or four pounds turned into ten or twenty, then I've gone too far out of sync. I've just smashed every wall and I need to rein myself back in. Same with alcohol—two or three beers isn't really going to hurt.

But 10 or 12 probably will.

The trick is to put everything into a box and be OK with allowing it to expand.

How far? That is up to you. It's up to your own judgment, but I know that when you start to think more about it, you'll know how far it is. As I mentioned in Chapter 2, you need to *think for yourself*. You don't need an app or to ask anyone else what their routine is. Find your own. If there's a bit of thought put into it, you'll find it will work nicely for how you want to live your life.

@THEPAULGOUGH

Six More Things To Consider in Pursuit of A Terrific Life

I agree in some ways that this work/life balance thing is important to consider. It's just more important that you consider what you really want from getting it.

As I always say, people don't want a successful business, they want to make money from it. And they don't even want the money, they want the *feeling* they think having the money will bring. The same can be said for work/life balance. People don't really dream about getting it. They want how they suppose it will make them feel.

In life, it's all about how you feel and as mentioned many times already, you are 100 percent in control of that, no matter what anyone tells you.

With that in mind, I'd like you to consider some other things that can shape how you feel about yourself and your life. In my humble opinion, they are just as important, if not more important to focus on, than the almighty work/life balance.

In fact, you could say that focusing on the following thoughts are what will really allow you to say you've got your house in order—that you are balanced and feel good about yourself—even if you don't make it home for dinner on time or decide to be at work for the next three weekends in a row.

These things are much less talked about than work/life balance in the entrepreneurial community, but, in my opinion, they're probably more important. In fact, I'd go out on a limb and suggest that if you *do* focus on these next six things, you'll probably be able to eradicate the need for any conversation about "work/life balance" from your life completely.

GET YOUR ACHIEVEMENT BOOK RESOURCE KIT: WWW.EXABOOK.COM/FREE

@THEPAULGOUGH

I believe the following are the *real* ingredients of a life that can be enjoyed and one that you feel good about living that might, just might, lead you to be able to say that you finally feel balanced.

1. Calmness

What's the point of working hard to buy an expensive car if you're always *angry* when you're driving home from work in it? You might have work/life balance, and you might be home for dinner on time, but what's the point if you're always angry and irate?

Personally, I think there's nothing worse than seeing successful people perpetually angry at the smallest of things, or always one conversation away from blowing their lid!

It's mostly a problem with expectations—the expectation that things *should* be different, that they *should* have not happened, or that they *should* have gone differently. It's the expectations that you bring to situations—and a bit of an overblown ego—that cause these frustrations.

I get it.

But really, nothing much in life is so important that you should ever give away your ability to live calm, cool, and collected, no matter if you're building a business or not.

If in doubt, remember this: It's OK to sweat the small stuff. Just because others get angry at trivial things, that doesn't mean you should. When people get angry at small stuff, it's a sign that their view of the world has also become small.

If it happens to you, which it inevitably will, take a deep breath, close your eyes, zoom out, and elevate yourself to the point where you're looking down on the world from as far above as you can possibly imagine. I've found doing so helps to really put into perspective how trivial and how insignificant whatever I am annoyed about really is.

Not long after, I calm down and I remind myself to smile and laugh at how seriously I was taking life.

2. Consistency

What's the point of having a million dollars in the bank if your kids don't know which version of Mom or Dad will walk through the door at night?

You might be at home for dinner—because you agreed to it as part of the work/life balance pact with your spouse—but who is really there?

Will it be the best version of Dad, or will it be the worst? Will it be Happy Mommy, or a mommy who lives within herself, always consumed by guilt about being at work in the first place? Is it the person who makes others feel amazing, or the one who always makes others feel like they've done something wrong?

I believe one of the greatest gifts you can ever give your kids is a feeling of being safe. And the only way to do that is to be *consistent*.

I lived with a parent who couldn't do this, so believe me when I tell you I learned this one the hard way. I have no doubt he loved me, but why did I feel so unsafe when he was around? It's because he wasn't *consistent* with his ability to control *his* emotions.

3. Contentment

What good is what you're doing if what you're achieving isn't making you more at ease with life and how you live it?

What good is being at your kid's football game as part of your work/life balance pact if you're living restlessly? What's the point in buying the massive house with the big swimming pool if you are not able to relax in it?

Tip: You can be *relentless* in your pursuit of entrepreneurial success. Just make sure it doesn't make you *restless*. The latter means you're never at ease with anything you do or achieve. And that type of life isn't worth living for any prize. It definitely isn't Extraordinary.

In fact, it's as *ordinary* as it gets, so common it is to see someone live this way. If you're going to focus on success, be sure to remind yourself that it doesn't and shouldn't come at the expense of never being content with you are.

If that doesn't work, I recommend you re-read Chapter 4, "What Drives You On Can Also Drive You Mad."

4. Confidence

Business—and life—are going to throw a lot of challenges and obstacles at you. What's the point of dealing with them all if they don't at the very least cause you to become a lot more confident about your life and how you live it?

Think about it. *What's the point?* Why would you not use the lessons you've taken and tests you've passed to enhance your life?

You can and should use the fact that you've overcome problems in life to grow your confidence in yourself so that as other problems *inevitably* come up, you're able to tackle them head on and with aplomb.

If you're not becoming more resilient and living with more conviction in your actions as a result of the journey you're on, why bother going on it? Stay at home and watch Netflix and eat pizza with everyone else. There's very little criticism from anyone during an episode of *Suits* or *House of Cards*. But there's also little in the way of feeling good about yourself and genuinely enjoying life.

Acknowledging that you can and have overcome adversity is how you build real confidence in yourself. Most people are *world class* at dealing with problems and making it through bad days. They just never take the time to realize it.

5. Centered

When people say they feel "off balance," it's happening because they are looking too far ahead—and always outside of themselves. The problem with looking too far into the future is that *psychological angst* appears in the gap the minute you do. The gap being the area between where you are now—the present—and a better future—the goal you imagined.

When you realize what you want in the future is in some way *better* than what you have or who you are today, that is when you become anxious and feel "off center." If you want to regain your balance, it's at that this precise moment—as you think about the future—that you have to catch yourself doing it and bring yourself back to today.

Sure, look into the future and have your grand vision, enjoy thinking about what life might be like or could be like in a year or so. Use it to inspire you. However, don't stay there. You can go there, but don't stay there. The trick is to bring everything back to today and then, crucially, accept that what you've got is already more than what you need.

That's what it means to *balance ambition with acceptance of yourself.* That thing I spoke about in the very first chapter of the book.

That's the journey that you're really on. One in which you embrace and relish commercial success but not at the expense of always thinking you're not good enough and getting it will make you better.

The trick is to remind yourself that everything in the future, while nice to have, it is not really needed. You want to get it or achieve it, but it's not much more than a sign that you've made a bit of progress in life. It's nothing that is going to make *you* better than you already are today.

Why is this important? It's because if you don't do this now, guess how you will feel when you get it (whatever *it* is)?

That's right. Exactly like you do now: that you're not good enough and that you need something else to fix it. On and on it goes. More and more work, yet another goal, rarely feeling any better despite hitting targets.

Sound familiar?

6. Compassion

To be a successful entrepreneur, you've got to learn a lot about yourself, business, life and the people in it. You've also got to grow a lot. It means you're going to have a very different perspective from most of the rest of the world, who aren't doing much of either—learning *or* growing.

Why is that a problem for you, you might ask?

Well, if you're not careful, you're going to drive yourself mad wondering why all the people around you don't see things as you do. To you, everything is going to be obvious, clear, and simple. To others, it's going to be difficult, murky, and impossible to achieve.

How you handle this is going to test every ounce of your compassion.

You're also going to *achieve* a lot. The problem is you are going to be living in a world with people who mostly, by their own private admission, haven't or never will. Sounds harsh, but it is true. Most aren't achieving what they thought they would, or living how they hoped, at this phase of their lives and their resentment toward other people's success gives you the biggest clue.

My tip to ensure you can co-exist without denying or covering up what you've achieved is to *act small* but never stop *thinking big*.

Don't go out of your way to parade your success in front of people, but equally, don't deny it either. If they don't ask you—don't tell them. It's that simple. But if they do ask about it, tell them. It isn't bragging if it's true.

Never shy away from what you've achieved and never feel guilty about it, just don't shout about it. If your success is permanently sat in the garage because you dare not drive it to the family party for fear of being judged, that's not right and you've still not achieved the thing you set out to do: accept yourself.

Most importantly, never lose sight of what you have achieved just because you're so focused on the fact that others haven't or don't acknowledge you for having done so. Their acknowledgement of your progress is nice, but mostly irrelevant and definitely not necessary.

When you started your business, the goal wasn't to get acknowledged by people—it was to give you and your family a terrific life and, as we mentioned earlier, to feel better about yourself.

Every single day *you* should acknowledge the fact that *you've done that* and watch how happy you become by doing so.

Major Principle of Chapter 12: Don't have too many hard deadlines or strict rules. Instead, give yourself permission to make real-time decisions and respond to things in your life as they occur.

ACHIEVEMENT
CHAPTER 13

Approval Not Needed

I often walk around town wearing a T-shirt *I made* with the words "Approval Not Needed" written across the front of it. It also has my signature below it to give it my own personal seal of approval. It's a reminder to myself of how I want to live my life and that is with the absolute belief that approval is not needed.

Not from anyone.

Not from my parents, my colleagues, my neighbors, my staff, or anyone else for that matter. They don't need my approval, why do I need theirs?

If there's one single thing I believe would *dramatically* alter the course of people's lives, for the better, it's the ability to live free from feeling judged, to be so secure and confident that you could do some "radical" things in your business like raise prices, fire miserable clients (and staff), and even pull up at the front door in a Ferrari with the personalized number plate "*Loaded 1*", and not care what your clients think of you for doing so.

I've touched on this earlier, but I firmly believe personal security is way more important than financial security. In fact, get the former, and it won't be that long before the latter arrives in your life as well.

If you took the "seeking approval" thing away from most people, the magic in their lives would really start to happen. It would certainly be dialled up a few notches.

That's because their *thoughts* would suddenly be different.

Rather than being consumed by worries about never being quite good enough, what they *lack*, or what they need to do to *impress*, in their place would be much more useful thoughts: ones of *possibility, opportunity, creativity, ambition,* and, above all else, how wonderful life and all that it can offer really is.

Life might be tough and a little unpredictable at times, but it's nothing if not abundant. The problem for most is simply that their *thinking* is quite the opposite. It's all about what is missing, what is lacking, and what is going to go wrong.

From never feeling like there's enough time in the day, or ever having had enough sleep, it's always about what wasn't or isn't there and it's no wonder most people live thinking the world is always conspiring against them. It's because their thoughts are telling them it is.

The feeling that you need to impress others is often impressed upon you from an early age. When you're seven and your mother wants you to do well in school—better than you want to do for yourself—you can't help but think you're going to let her down if you don't.

Because of that, you set about working that little bit harder. It's not *just* to be good in school and to get good grades, it's mostly to please Mother. Let's face it, at seven, you have no idea why doing well in English is even that important.

You get on and do the work and then later, when your mother tells you something like, "I'm so happy you did well on your English test," and you see *that* smile on her face, you make the link between your actions and someone else's happiness. If you're not careful, it's also the end of living *your* life as you know it. That's because you then carry that feeling with you all your life.

And what feeling is that?

The one that has you believe that other people are depending upon you to feel better. It's fine when you're doing well. Like in school, when you're seven and pass a simple test and bring your report card home. However, what about when the inevitable happens and you start to struggle or fail at a few things?

What happens then? How do you react when what you do doesn't please?

Because you made the link between your success and others being happy, you can't help but feel bad about yourself at the thought you've let others down. It's why so many people put enormous pressure on themselves to do things, even if they don't make them happy. It's mostly to *please others*.

And what about *that day* that arrives in all our lives—the one where you want to live a different life than the one your parents planned for you?

How does that play out if you think your parents are relying upon you to get married at a certain age, or go to college to get a certain degree, to allow you to enter a certain type of profession, one that *they* approve of? What happens then when you buck their trend?

Well, I'll tell you what happens. It's usually one of two things:

You go your own way and live your own life but then spend the rest of it worrying that you let someone down (basically, riddled with *guilt* and *regret*).

You become a perpetual *people pleaser*, regretting that you didn't get to live your own life, always resenting the fact no matter what you do, no one seems to be grateful or appreciate the choices you made.

If I was to hazard a guess, I'd say most people choose the second option. And if you have done anything like that, you're not alone. There are millions, if not billions, of "people pleasers" all over the world, most of them struggling to ever live a day of their *own life,* and all in the name of trying to make someone else happy.

But here's the thing I often think about: is it just about pleasing someone else? In a nice way, where you do so because you want them to feel good knowing you caused it? Or does so much people pleasing happen because so many people *lack the courage* to say no to doing it?

I suspect it's a bit of both. People like to make others feel good—it's a fast route to feeling good yourself sort tern—but there's also at least a *bit* of truth to the idea that it exposes a lack of courage in how people live.

"I'm a People Pleaser"

@THEPAULGOUGH

I always find it funny when people talk about themselves as a "people pleaser." There are so many who claim to do it, or be one, yet so many people in the world remain unhappy. It means there are either a lot of *incompetent* people pleasers out there or a lot of very hard-to-please people walking the planet.

A bit of both, perhaps?

On a serious note, people pleasing is a big thing in society. It's a badge of honor that people love to give themselves. And yes, as I write these words, I am acutely aware of the many thousands of people who at this precise moment are screaming, "*This is me*! I'm a people pleaser—I've been doing it all my life!"

People pleasing, although admirable, must be one of the most frustrating things you can ever try to do. It's the fast route to living unsatisfied, disappointed, and probably a little angry that no matter what you do, people don't seem to value you as much as you deserve.

Can you relate?

If so, the trick to breaking free from being a perpetually frustrated people pleaser, to just being *pleased with yourself*, is to first accept that *you* alone can't please people. It requires that the other person is even capable of being pleased, and that's a big assumption to make.

The other part you must know is how people pleasers become people pleasers. It happens because they *think* they're letting others down if they don't conform or behave a certain way.

Although it's easy to think that way, the truth is this: it's not you letting them down, it's *them* letting *themselves* down.

That's because anyone who is expecting you to do things to make them happy or feel better about themselves has in fact let *themselves* down.

Unknowingly, unwittingly, unconsciously—whatever word you want to use for having no clue they did so—they've *absolved* themselves of their number one job in life, and that is their *own* responsibility to make *themselves* happy and feel better through their *own* thoughts and actions. It's a duty that each of us has and can never be outsourced.

You can outsource your laundry, your admin, your marketing, and a few other things—but not your responsibility for making yourself happy. You show me anyone who is chronically unhappy, not to mention insecure, and I'd bet the farm they've outsourced their happiness to someone else.

Here's the thing to remember: if someone wants you to live *their* version of *your* life, it's because they've told themselves that this is the pathway to *them* feeling better.

So confused are they about what they need from their life, and how to feel better about their life, that they come to the bizarre conclusion that you must behave exactly how they say you should. It's nuts, it doesn't make any sense, but it'll keep happening largely because people seem to think that finding someone else to make them happy is the goal of life.

How can knowing this help you?

There are two ways, and they're both simple.

The first is to make sure that you never live this way. Make sure that *you* never outsource the responsibility for your happiness to someone else. Not to your partner, your kids, or anyone else, ever. Don't burden people any more than they already are with their own issues.

And the second is that knowing all of this allows you to have a bit of detachment from what others are thinking or expecting of you and, possibly, even a little bit of compassion for anyone who does expect you to jump on demand. Turn your incessant need to please into the real need to understand people's inability to please themselves.

Basically, change the *meaning* of it all.

If you're currently feeling like you're being judged by your parents, your partner, your employees, or anyone else, never forget that judgement is a **weakness in their life—not yours.** It's a weakness that you will never fix, no matter how much you do or what level of success you achieve. They'll always need more from you.

In fact, in the end, they could even come to resent just how successful you've become on your way to pleasing them. It really is screwed up, but don't allow yourself to become a surrogate drug for their happiness in life—no matter how much you love them.

My tip is to love them enough to let them figure out how to make themselves happy. It'll be the best thing you can ever do for *anyone*.

Never forget that you can be a good, kind, caring person and *still* say no to people, prioritize your needs, set boundaries, disagree, be candidly honest, and walk away from toxic environments. You can also make mistakes, challenge poor behavior, and protect your time and space, not to mention your feelings, and it doesn't say anything about you other than perhaps you've got enough self-respect and control of your own mind to do so.

Only jealous, or very *insecure*, people who want to make you feel bad about yourself would tell you otherwise.

And by the way, if they want or try to make you feel like that, ask yourself why anyone with your best interests at heart would do that. Then ask what the heck they're doing in your life in the first place.

Why Perfectionists Get Nothing Done

While we're on the subject of *insecure people*, now is a perfect time to talk about *perfectionists*. No *pun* intended. There are millions of so called, self labeled perfectionists out there and as you'll soon see, it pays to know how to spot them or avoid trying to be like one.

If nothing else, it can be quite the hinderance to entrepreneurial success. It'll definitely stop you from getting to the next level.

I'll start by saying perfectionists are a clever bunch.

They are the most insecure people on the planet, and they get nothing done, but somehow they manage to pull the wool over many people's eyes about how wonderful they are and how "perfect" they are at, well, everything. They even have people wanting to emulate them. Me included.

As a kid, I used to be impressed with perfectionists. I used to look up to and admire them and I would often consider how to become one, so convinced was I that being a perfectionist was a worthwhile pursuit.

However, no matter how hard I tried, I just couldn't reach perfection. I guess I wasn't cut out for a life of excuses and procrastinating, so off I went back to my life of things being less than perfect but getting stuff done and making progress regardless.

No regrets, either.

So *why do* perfectionists get nothing done?

Well, let me tell you: It's because they dare not put out to the world what they've done for fear of criticism they can't handle. The project is always being "worked on," it's always "nearly finished" and "not quite ready" because they know that they cannot handle how they will feel if the work is scorned.

On and on the stalling goes, always waiting until "it's perfect," always hoping to avoid the criticism they fear not being able to handle, and it's all in the name of it being "perfect."

It highlights the biggest issue in their lives: they lack the ability to deal with the idea that other people think badly of them. They are an unconscious victim of their own need to be perfect, and the lack of progress or constant fear they live with is the penalty they will pay.

I've hired a few "perfectionists" in my office and eventually I came to conclusion that they all had the same thing in common: *nothing*. That is, they all produced *nothing*.

I've discovered a few other things about perfectionists, too.

One big one is that perfectionists can't wait to tell you they're a perfectionist. It's often the first thing they'll tell you when you ask why they haven't done anything despite sitting in their seat for a week.

What is funny is they say it as though I am going to be impressed. They genuinely think it's going to be something I'm happy to hear.

However, they're usually less than impressed with my response. I tell them I have no time for perfectionists and that they're in the wrong job working for the wrong boss if that's who they are. I remind them that their job only exists because I prioritize getting things *done* over things being perfect (and non-existent) and I tell them bluntly that *possible is better than perfect*.

And that is the mantra I would encourage you to take with you on your entrepreneurial journey: *possible is better than perfect*.

It is one thing to be a perfectionist if you're an employee of a company that is so big it doesn't notice you're not getting much done, or you work for a boss who's not clever enough to understand what your self-imposed label really means for his or her bottom line.

But if you're an entrepreneur and you're claiming to be a perfectionist, that's a complete disaster. It's just not in the job description of a CEO. Not only will you not get anything done, you'll also breed that "must be perfect" mindset throughout your company. It means there'll be lots of "working on it" and "a few weeks away from finishing it," but little in the way of results.

The key to getting things done is to be comfortable with the consequences of them not being perfect. It's to find the balance between not needing approval of your work but at the same time accepting that enough people do need to like it for it to produce the results you want.

The trick is to find what is called the "good enough spot."

One of the simple differences between someone like me who gets a lot done and a perfectionist who gets very little done is that I work toward the "good enough spot," or GE spot, with everything I do. It might not be perfect, but it's good enough. And good enough is good enough as far as I am concerned.

Besides, the GE spot is also much *easier to find.*

Anyway, because I can deal with criticism, laugh off the comments on Facebook, and even handle the emails about spelling mistakes in my emails or blogs, it means I can put my work out faster than others. And given that "speed to market" is a prerequisite of success in entrepreneurship, this ability gives me a massive advantage over others still "working on it."

But what does it all really matter when you get down to it anyway?

If it's not "perfect", so what?

Seriously, who made up the rule that the odd spelling mistake matters anyway? Your English language teacher? Your parents? Or is the people whose lives are so empty that they're triggered by the spelling mistake in the first place?

I find it quite funny that people get so irate over a spelling mistake or two.

It is a reminder to me of how *serious* others take life and I thank my lucky stars I'm not one of them. It also highlights which clients I'd like to work with and let's just say it's not the ones who point out a spelling mistake, that's for sure.

The occasional spelling mistake doesn't mean I'm a complete failure or the worst writer England ever produced. I have more spelling mistakes in my emails and marketing material than anyone else I know—but here you are, reading my sixth best-selling book!

If it were left to conventional wisdom and societal rules, such a thing would not happen to a writer with such a tendency for misspelling words. But like I've maintained throughout this book, conventional wisdom is usually far from wise.

What's ironic is that when I was fifteen years old, my English language teacher told my mother at a parents evening that I would fail my exam as I "wasn't a very good writer."

It's a true story.

She told my mother that she should expect an "D" in my test—maybe a "C" if I was having a good day. As the story goes, I ended up with an "A" in English language and a "B" in English literature.

I would love to write and tell my ex-teacher that she was obviously a better teacher than she gave herself credit for, and perhaps send her a copy of all of my best sellers. But I don't hold out much hope that it would make a difference in her opinion of me. She seemed pretty convinced that I was a bad student who couldn't write.

Besides, I don't think Amazon delivers to the cemetery.

Anyhow, I digress. I want you to remember from this little section that possible is better than perfect. As an entrepreneur with *ambition* to grow a successful business, you are going to have to get things done fast and not all of it will be perfect when it needs to be launched. *Not* being able to handle criticism about imperfection is a sure-fire way to guarantee you won't get anything done and therefore stay stuck.

A simple, almost instantaneous way to find a little more belief in yourself is to remind yourself daily that everyone else suffers from a lack of belief in themselves as well.

Remember that the ones who are judging you and your work are doing so because it's a break from the incessant worrying about never being good enough themselves. It's a break from feeling low. Complaining about you stops the criticism of themselves that they've never found any other way to do.

Seriously, a simple way to beat insecurity is it to understand that this insecurity thing *isn't* just happening to you. Look into the eyes of everyone you meet today and if you look long enough, it won't be long before *they* wonder if *you* are seeing right through *them* and right into the soul of who they are: people who are insecure worried about being exposed.

Basically, it means we're all a bit screwed up, but the person who knows it and accepts it has a chance of being a bit less screwed up than the rest. *Lovely.*

When in doubt, remember that they're not thinking about you at all. No. They're doing what you are doing—worrying about *themselves* and how they appear to *you*.

If you can hold your nerve for just long enough to remember this, you won't find yourself in too many situations where you feel less valuable, less worthy, or beneath the person you're talking to. The key is to stare right into their eyes and hold the glare.

When you do, you'll notice most can't look at you for longer than a few seconds before they start to worry about what it is you're seeing.

Non-Negotiables: The Foundation for a Great Life

One of the best things you can do to find more belief in yourself is to better *understand* yourself. I believe the more you realize about yourself, the more you can back yourself. The more that you know to be true about yourself, the easier it is to live consistently with what you say you want.

Basically, the deeper understanding that you have about who you really are, the more confidence you have in who you are and what you are about.

Could it be true that most people don't really know themselves all that well and that's why they're never able to get what they want *or* feel how they want?

Again, I don't know for sure. But I suspect there's at least *some* truth to that.

Take the time to get clear on precisely what you want for yourself and how you are willing to live your life and I'll go out on a limb and suggest you'll immediately live with more purpose and intention. It'll definitely feel as though life is more of what you might call "your own." How novel.

Now what I am talking about here are things you might call "non-negotiables."

They are the bedrock of your actions and thoughts, and the foundation for your decisions in the busyness of day-to-day life. These are things that you will staunchly refuse to negotiate on, so valuable and important they are to you living your life, on your terms.

Here are a few examples of the non-negotiables in my life to give you some inspiration for creating your own:

1. I must be doing work that energizes me

People say that I'm a guy with a lot of energy, but if you put me into a role that I'm not in love with, you might find that I'm not playing at the same level. My energy doesn't come from sleep or food, it is primarily from my work. I make it my goal to only do work that energizes me. And ideally, pays me the most money.

2. I must be working with people I enjoy working with

I have a simple but important rule in my life—no moaning. I can't stand people who moan with no intention of changing whatever it is they're moaning about. I always say that you can *rant*, *vent*, or *let off steam* around me, but if you're still making the same noise about the same thing days later, and you haven't done something about it, you are moaning. And that's not cool. It's certainly something I am not willing to accept or tolerate for too long.

3. The effort must be worth the reward

If I'm committing my days and energy to something, it must be *really* worth it. It can't just be for the sake of it or for marginal gains. If I am giving my energy, I want a big reward for doing so. I have no intention of spending my life committed to a cause that isn't worth it in terms of the things I can do, places I go, and the standard of living I can achieve for me and my family.

4. **My work week and calendar is 100% controlled by me**

I always want to decide how my week looks, including when I'll work and when I'll be on vacation. If I can't do that, or people want me to do things that disrupt my family or personal time, I won't get involved in it.

Side note: this wasn't always the case in the early days of building my business, but I recommend getting there as fast as you can. You'll never feel like you're ready to this though, and the only way to be ready is to find the courage to do it even though you're not (you might need to re-read that, but it's worth understanding.)

5. I must be able to travel frequently and enjoy extended vacations uninterrupted (minimum six to eight weeks off and unplugged per year)

I love to travel extensively and doing so is *the* source of a lot of my ideas, creativity, and motivation. It's a major part of my life and extended vacations and travel time is the reward for what I do. It's not a break from it when I'm burnt out like it is for so many.

I like author Tim Ferris's view on this: why wait until you retire to travel the world? I like lots of mini vacations and I suspect they will push back my desire to retire in the first place.

6. Success cannot come at the price of my health

If something is costing me my health—via stress, anxiety, etc.—it needs to be stopped immediately and I'm prepared to pull the plug on pretty much anything or anyone that causes it.

I am the source of all the good things that spawn from the work I do, and I must protect my health (and my thinking!) in the same way that a top basketball team would protect its best players. In the same way that injured basketball players can't score points, unhealthy business owners can't make money.

7. Nothing can be so important that I need to be reached any time day or night

Most people thrive on the idea that they can be reached at any time, day or night. Personally, I couldn't think of anything worse. Like I said in an earlier chapter on distractions, having a phone and being accessible 24/7 is not conducive of a productive of enjoyable life. I set my life up, business included, whereby I don't ever have to answer the phone unplanned.

I value my own time, my own thoughts, not to mention the conversations I am having with others in person, more than I do being accessible 24/7. If there's an emergency, you can call my office, or Natalie, and they'll pass the message on to me. I'll get back to you at a pre-arranged time.

So there you go…those are just a *few* of the non-negotiables that I have at this point of my life. I'm not saying that you need seven, or that any of these are right or wrong. They're simply right for me——right now.

I recommend you spend some time thinking about your own list and then, most importantly of all, actually *live* the items on your list! Don't put them up on the wall, on a fancy canvas for everyone to see and then pay lip service to them.

If you say you want to be uncontactable during the evening or at the weekend, put your phone in the freezer after work or, better yet, insist that your staff call your partner to get to you. That should make them think twice before calling you to tell you the coffee machine is broken and ask what to do about it.

Anyway, let's move on to the next chapter and talk about another way to solve the insecurity problem and fix any need you're living with to feel approval.

Major Principle of Chapter 13: Approval is not needed from anyone, perfectionists get nothing done, and people pleasing is futile. Put an end to it all.

ACHIEVEMENT
CHAPTER 14

The Ultimate Investment

A few years ago, I bought an iPad from the Apple Store. At the same time, I was asked if I would like to spend an additional $100 or so on five sessions with a "genius" who would teach me how to understand and navigate the operating system of said iPad. It made sense to me to spend a bit of money to learn how to use something I'd just spent a lot of money on.

I paid my money and off I went, attending my five sessions across five weeks with a "genius" at a store in Santa Monica, California.

While there, I was a little surprised by just how many people were doing the same thing: spending money with a "genius" to learn how to use the same device or similar as I had bought.

At the sight of so many people attending the lessons with these "geniuses"—often twenty-one-year-old college kids dropped off at work by their parents—I couldn't help but wonder just how many of the hundreds of people spending $100 with an Apple "genius" would ever spend the same amount on figuring out their own operating system—that being *their own minds*.

See, it isn't just the Apple iPad that has a unique operating system that can do amazing things—*all* humans have one too.

The problem is very few people are willing to invest time and money into learning how to use it. And that's what I believe is causing most people's frustration in life. It's not a lack of opportunity, it's a lack of understanding on how to use their own supercomputer for the purpose of enhancing and aiding a good quality of life.

I've heard it said that the root of all stress is a lack of knowledge.

I believe that is at least *somewhat* true.

For example, and like I said in Chapter 4, most business owners live with stress and angst and it's often because of an incessant need to prove to their parents they're good enough. They lack knowledge on the real, root cause of the issue and so attempt to fix it by making more money. A bottle of red wine and a weekly therapy session *might* relieve the pain temporarily, but it does nothing to fix the demons once and for all.

Only seeking out real knowledge, about the real problem, can do that. That takes an investment of time, and often money, and they are things that people seem to find any excuse to avoid making.

It's sad but true that very few, if any, people are willing to spend time and money on learning how to use the operating system they are born with, let alone developing it. It is assumed that the passage of time or some "life experience" —whatever that is—is all a person needs to better understand himself.

Except it isn't. And I'll give you a few common scenarios to prove it.

That guy or girl who *always* gets angry at the same thing, day after day, has a lack of *understanding* why it's happening. That guy or girl who is on to their fourth relationship, never able to trust anyone, always thinking it's the *other* person's fault, doesn't *understand* why *they're* so insecure and possibly causing every relationship to break down because of that, and is refusing to learn.

That entrepreneur who can't commit to getting anything done, despite having the best of intentions, doesn't *understand* why doubt creeps in every time they start something.

That entrepreneur who can't trust staff and *still* struggles with delegation ten years later doesn't understand where the need for everything to be perfect comes from, and is refusing to learn.

That same entrepreneur who can't let people make decisions and do their jobs, despite having twenty people on payroll, can't understand why they can't let go of control.

It's very easy to blame life's circumstances, but the *real* reason people are stuck at the level they are is because they lack an understanding of why they're there in the first place and only the pharmaceutical companies stand to benefit from this.

If people knew the real cause of their problem, they wouldn't be as stressed or depressed there wouldn't be a need for pills to relieve it.

Of course, I can't prove that. But I do have a strong hunch!

If nothing else, remember this: the level of life people are at is often a reflection of their thinking and that is often a reflection of their commitment to themselves to be a well-rounded individual.

That includes the emotional, spiritual, financial, and physical aspects of life.

It's easy to commit to a gym and improve how you look physically. Not so easy to pick up a book or hire a coach to improve how you *think*. After all, no one is going to comment on how *great your thinking* is like they do an improved physique.

Life Like A Hollywood Movie

If you've picked up on my contrarian view of life, my resentment toward the political and modern-day education system, or why I don't think taxing the rich will ever change anything, it's because of this one single thing: I firmly believe the only way to make any real, sustainable difference in your life is to invest your own *time* and often *money* into discovering more about yourself and learning what makes you tick. That is where the personal security that people crave really comes from.

Yet, if you look at most people's lives, it's the complete opposite.

They will know which celebrity has gone into rehab and can tell you who the guy over the road is having an affair with, but they'll not be able to tell you why they're so *fearful* about life and are always consumed by guilt and regret.

They think it's normal, that it must be that way, and they hope that one day, perhaps when they win the lottery, it'll all go away, and life will *finally* be like what they've seen in those pretentious Hollywood movies.

The cruel irony of life is we are all born with the potential to do more and create more than anything else on the planet. The computer that sits in our heads is capable of so much, but the big problem—perhaps irony?—is it does not come with a set of lessons on how to use it. It's a bit like buying a 30,000-piece LEGO set that is missing the instructions.

The picture on the front of the box looks amazing, but there's no way to piece it together without a lot of mistakes and frustration. Investing in yourself is the equivalent of getting the instructions and ridding yourself of the mistakes and frustration that inevitably come with building the LEGO set without them.

And that, I believe, is a metaphor that sums up life in the twenty-first century.

The images we see on social media or that are sold to us by the "elders" in society are stunning. We're all told we can be anything and do anything we want, but there are no instructions given at birth on how to make that a reality. And because not many people you talk to have figured it out either, it's a case of the blind leading the blind, each person hoping the one they're copying has it figured out.

In essence, it means most people are using the iPad without any clue how to work it properly. At best, they are being taught by failed iPad users how to use the iPad successfully.

The sad fact of the society that we live in is that people dare not, will not, and simply are not comfortable with investing in themselves over and above what they receive in mainstream education.

Which, I might add, does very little but raise expectations for success in life. Mainstream education is expensive, it takes time, and it is an investment of sorts, but it does little to equip people with the tools to be happy, fulfilled, and able to live at the next level of life, with a lot more money than they need before rent day comes around again.

How *dare* I say this?

Because there are millions of people passing through the same system: preschool to school, school to college, then on to university and into a job, meaning there are millions of people coming out with that $100,000 certificate in something like *historical biology*, or *archaeological politics*, or whatever, and yet here we are, millions of people in unstainable debt, stuck in unhappy marriages and living life without the feeling of control.

Certainly these are not the lives people *assumed* they would get when they enrolled or signed the check for that fancy out-of-state college.

Is the education system broke?

Of course not. It's one of the richest organizations in the world.

Does it work at producing happy, fulfilled, content, and rich individuals, all equipped with the skills necessary to handle real life, and embrace the challenges and uncertainty it brings? Absolutely not. And for that reason, if you ask me, it is broken.

That's why the investment in mainstream education isn't the only one you need to make. And especially not if you're an entrepreneur. There are very few people at college who can teach you how to run profitable business. If they could, they wouldn't be picking up a teacher's salary. They'd be out there doing it for themselves and making a few million or so for themselves.

They definitely wouldn't be hanging around for job security and the promise of a decent retirement fund.

"How Did I Do It?"

@THEPAULGOUGH

If you asked me to describe my life, I'd do so using one word—*different!* Different in how I think, different in how I live, not to mention different in the opportunities and things that are available to me in comparison to the majority of the world and people around me.

I'm not for one second suggesting that my life is perfect, or in any way better, but it is undeniably different and I've definitely done and continue to do a lot of things that others are trying to do and yet, I reckon I've been asked *how I did* it by no more than two or three people (aside from clients I consult with, that is).

I sit next to friends and family with debt problems, or with issues in their businesses, and the same people tell me how hard life is, how tough it is and how unhappy they are with what they've got, but rarely does any of them ever ask, "How did you sort your house out Paul?"

See, I think most people look at my life and if they know anything about it they *assume* it is all achieved by luck, or that I was born with a permanent smile on my face and the divine gift of being able to make money so easily you'd be forgiven for thinking I have a printing press in my home. None of that is true.

If you got close to me, and you asked me, "Paul, how did you get the life you've got today, with so many *choices* and so much *fun* in it?" I'd look you dead in the eye and tell you straight it's because I *took a risk* and invested in myself beyond the investment required of organized education or that of an hour with an Apple "genius."

Simple, really.

@THEPAULGOUGH

It's not that I'm a rocket scientist or have "genius" level IQ reserved for top doctors, lawyers, or inventors. I did OK in school, but I knew I wasn't *that* clever. I passed all of my exams, but I definitely wasn't a genius.

However, I was clever enough to realize that I didn't need to be one of those to live a great life. I don't know how, but I realized early that there was something more to life than following society's rules and scraping by, and instead, I sought a life that is more about personal growth and expansion and I was curious enough to want to see what life was like beyond the level I had grown up with.

As an aside, even the commonly accepted view of a *genius* is messed up and causing a lot of people to remain stuck.

Society has done a wonderful job of putting certain people and careers on a lofty pedestal and making you think you've got to be some sort of genius to get there. Although easy to accept, the truth is that being a "genius" is not so much about intelligence but simply the *ability* to put into effect what is in your mind.

Sure, there are a few people with a high level of intelligence who you might consider geniuses. But for the most part, the people you admire and perhaps would be forgiven for labelling geniuses are not always of Einstein-level intelligence. Instead, they are everyday people with a reasonable level of intelligence who figured out how to take what was in their heads and turn it into reality.

That's it. Mystery over. Something that almost everyone reading this book is capable of, if they so choose. A bit like being *extra*ordinary—it's simply ordinary with a few extras. You just need to realize how simple it is to achieve.

@THEPAULGOUGH

The real issue for most entrepreneurs is *not* that they lack genius—we each have a genie in us waiting to be rubbed and released. It's that they struggle to do what they say they will. This is also the chief reason for their lack of confidence. Another misconstrued idea is that people are either born with confidence or not. It's another limiting label they give themselves. "I've never been the confident type" is the mantra.

But truth is, no one is born with it.

If you ask me, it is *learned* and *earned*.

Learned in that as you invest more in yourself, you develop a superior knowledge on a particular subject compared to other people you're talking to. This becomes evident when you talk. And *earned* in that you make and subsequently keep promises to yourself that others do not.

A major reason most people lack confidence is because they've let themselves down so many times before. They are not a victim of biology or DNA; they are a culprit of their own inability to do something they said they would but couldn't make happen. Like the perfectionist, and the people pleaser, they're unconsciously trapped in that way of living and a lack of confidence is the hall mark.

It can all start with something as simple as, "I will get up and go to the gym at 6 AM tomorrow." Many say it. Yet, when that alarm goes off the snooze button is hit every nine minutes for two hours. Do this type of thing often enough and you lose faith in yourself to ever do anything you say you will.

In the end, this becomes the story of life, and your life becomes a victim of its reality: that you *won't* do what you say you will. I believe the difference between a genius and everyone else—especially in the context of entrepreneurship—is being able to make things happen than others can't. It's doing things that others can't or won't.

And one of those things is *investing in yourself*.

The best entrepreneurs are comfortable investing in learning about themselves, in understanding themselves and the commercial needs of their businesses in the same way the best athletes are comfortable investing time and money into their bodies and fitness. In that way, they match their intuition with facts and truths.

They don't rely on "gut instinct" like so many others do who then later blame that same gut when they get yet another decision wrong.

Over the years I've invested so much time and money into educating myself and developing myself that I can, without any hesitation, tell you that the life I'm living today is all *bought and paid for*. It wasn't handed down or given to me on a platter. It was bought. Or invested in, whichever way you want to see it.

Sure, there have been a few lucky breaks. But guess what? We all get them. The difference is I was ready when all of them came my way. Success happens when preparation meets opportunity. If you're ready, and you're looking, success shows up not long after.

As I think about my life, it's clear that everything significant happened because I was ready for it and that happened because I took a chance long before I even knew what the opportunity was. It's why I believe that the stars do not align looking forward, only looking *backward*.

You make the commitment, then you put your faith in the process, the universe, good things happening to intentional people, or whatever, and hope that all the things you took a shot at come together somehow, at some point, when you need it most.

And it's been my experience that they usually *do*.

I don't always know when, or where, or how, but eventually, the stars align, and each star is somehow connected to one before.

When you sign up for that marketing seminar, you won't know for certain there is someone there you want to meet. You have to sign up hoping that will happen. You've got to get up in the middle of the night, take that lonely flight to the other side of the world, and simply hope that when you return it will have been worth it.

Likewise, you can't invest in the business coach when you're certain you are ready, you must invest to get ready. There's a difference.

People Are Waiting, *Always* Waiting...

And that's another thing I've observed. Most people are never ready for anything. That's the real story of their life, all their life: waiting, always waiting. They're never ready to do the thing that would get them ready for how they want to feel.

They're always waiting for the day they feel better, or more confident, but it never comes because it's *at* the seminar, or working *with* the business coach, or being *in* that peer group or mastermind, etc., that they get that feeling they need.

They must do those things to *become* the person they want to be, but they won't. They're hoping it'll change with time or age, good fortune, a winning lottery ticket, or a piece of a large inheritance left by Daddy.

@THEPAULGOUGH

As I look at my life, I can tell you that it's worked out the way it's worked out because I *got* ready to *be* ready. COVID arrived and had most business owners panicking. Yet, to me, it was the situation I had been in training for, for more than a decade. While others panicked, I picked up my business plan, ripped it up, and made a new one in less than an hour, never worrying once that things wouldn't be OK.

"Why would it not be OK?" I would often ask Natalie.

I'd done the work *years before* on how to deal with uncertainty and live with risk, and I knew just how to change a marketing plan and sales process to suit the current needs of my clients. I'd invested in my personal and business skills and this was the time to use them. As a result, the only thing I had to worry about during COVID was the effect on my health should I catch it, and not the effect it would have on my business or family life. That was always going to be OK.

I made the ultimate decision to invest in myself and that took me to places to learn things and meet new people and those people helped me during situations I didn't even know were going to happen. Like COVID. I know I could never be doing what I am doing or living how I am without doing so.

Sure, at first, when I was spending money on my education and personal development it felt risky, scary, and, yes, it was very difficult to explain to others why I was doing it or what I was getting from it.

Many times, I didn't know myself. But I did it anyway. I came back from one seminar having met someone who *two years later* had an answer to a business challenge in my life, or met someone who introduced me to someone else I should connect with at the next event, all the while developing my network of people playing at the level I wanted to be at.

I bought courses with the profits of one business that I used to start the next business when others would have bought a new car. I used my spare time to read books that contained information I didn't even know I needed to know when others were at the bar watching football.

One book led me to the next book to find the answers to the questions raised from reading the last one. On and on it went. Always creating stars that would later align, getting ready for an opportunity, or crisis in the case of COVID, that I didn't know was coming.

Anyway, here I am, today, living a life that makes no sense to most people, and yet most people would like a slice of it. Especially the part where I'm able to live so freely, going places and getting there however I so choose, doing things as and when I wish, for as long as I wish.

Basically, I have a life that knows very few limits.

One thing I love about my life is how confused people are about what I do these days. I swear that Natalie's parents think I'm a drug dealer or that I've won the lottery and not announced it. They're definitely a bit perplexed about why I don't treat patients at my physical therapy clinic anymore—despite being a physical therapist who owns a physical therapy clinic! I've given up trying to explain.

Is my life perfect? Of course not.

Like I said back in Chapter 1, I'm a work in progress.

Is it all clear sailing? *Nope.* Life keeps on tossing things at me I am not yet ready to deal with but because of the investment I've made in myself, I am able to better deal with them. And by better, I mean less emotional. *Shit still happens*, but I can deal with anything unexpected in a way that allows me to keep moving *despite* not always wanting to be in the situation I am in. It's where all my progress really comes from.

And it's the same for you.

All *your* future progress comes from being able to get up faster after being hit; from being able to make decisions even though you don't feel ready; from being able to deal with situations and even setbacks that weren't necessarily your fault but happened anyway. That's what will separate you from the rest: the ability to do things even though you don't feel ready for them. That's another step on the path to an extraordinary life.

I made the ultimate investment, in myself, and because of that I'm living with real freedom in my life, absent of false responsibilities and with more than a touch of that *joie de vivre* I mentioned earlier in the book. I've got lot more cash available to me these days too. Which is nice. Especially as I've developed a bit of a love of traveling on a private jet. Not good for global warming, I know, but great for avoiding the mess that is TSA.

If you ask me what I am most proud of in my life, it's not the money, or the things and stuff in it, it's that *I* created it.

It's that I created a truly unique life that isn't following anyone else's design or expectations. I found my own path and followed it. It's why I struggle to explain to people what I do—there are very few frames of reference. At best I might be able to say something like *I used to make people healthy, now I make them rich, and best of all I get to enjoy the process of doing it.*

What I wish for you is that you get to find your own unique path, too.

That *you* become a truly unique self-creation. That you one day struggle to explain to people what you do and laugh when they ask you to explain it again, or better yet, pretend they understand when they obviously don't.

I want you to live knowing that you're proud of yourself for the life you created, without justifying your actions to anyone, living courageously enough to get what you want despite what others might think, ending up with more than enough left over to share it with the people close to you.

It would be so easy to say I'm proud of all the patients I've helped feel better when I was a physical therapist, or the clients whose businesses and lives are now improved by my marketing company. I am, of course I am, but all of that was only made possible *because* of the work I did on myself first.

If I was able to help them all, it's because I sorted myself out first. It's because I put my own seat belt on first. And if I've been able to help you in any way (through this book perhaps?) it's because I helped myself first. That's why I say I'm proud of myself for what I've created. I did it all. I got off my ass and went for it!

Yes, I've had unbelievable support from Natalie and people like my mother and my sister, my grandparents and cousins, *some* of my staff, even my father in the early days.

But I was the one who got out of bed at 4 AM to take that flight to the *first* marketing seminar in another country with a ticket paid for with my own money that kickstarted it all for me.

Ultimately it was me who took all the risks. It's the way it had to be. No one else could take the risks for me, only I could do that and I believe that's why the rewards arrive. They're directly proportional to the level of risk that you take.

It worked for me and it's the going to be the same for you. All of your future success will happen because of the risks you take today.

"You Won't Get Out Alive"

While we're on the subject of risk, I am 100 percent convinced that fear of **failing in the eyes of the world is the single biggest impediment to making real money from business**. It's the biggest risk and it stops most people dead in their tracks.

Yet, if you cannot crack this, you will always struggle to live at the level you so desire. This alone is the biggest difference I see between the people who make it to where they want and the rest.

The problem for most people is they can't live with the *risk of losing their money*.

They are so enslaved to it that they can't bear the thought of it ever going to waste. It's fine if it is wasted on alcohol and gambling, and the like, but not on a couple hours with a business coach, just in case.

And yet, all riches are found in the ability to live with the ability to manage risk. You simply cannot get rich—monetarily or in quality of life—without taking a risk or two.

I like Tony Robbins's take on this: "It's risky out there. So risky that you're not going to make it out alive." A simple way of saying that life is one big risk and no matter how much you try, it'll get you in the end no matter how much you hide away.

Might as well enjoy until then, don't you think?

I'm sure it's easy for people to look at me and say, "It's OK for you, Paul, you have the money to invest in yourself."

And I always respond, "Yes, that's why I have the money— because I did".

I found a way of putting more money into *myself* than a clothes store or car garage, and the returns soon became so large that spending tens of thousands every year on myself with a mentor or business coach became easier.

It was as simple as investing a small amount, getting a return, investing a bit more, getting a bit more back, investing a lot more, getting a lot more back, and so on. On and on it went until life and what I could get from it became more than I'd ever dreamed.

It's why I tell anyone it's really easy to get ahead in life. Just be willing to do the thing most aren't and that is *spend money on your own personal and business development*.

Might you have to pay a thousand dollars or so to start the process? Yes. But that shouldn't spook you. It's the deal. It's the thing that'll separate you from the ones who speak ambition but never achieve it.

Just a few weeks before writing this chapter, I flew to Cleveland, Ohio, to spend a day with a long-time business consultant who over the years has helped me tremendously.

I told a friend how much the day cost me—flights, hotel, and day with mentor all rounded up, I didn't get much change from $30,000. I was with him for *six* hours.

When I told my friend, he nearly choked on his drink.

He said to me, "That's expensive!"

I replied, "Relative to what?" Spending the next 30 years of my life making an average salary and living an average life, when I could spend it making a multi-million-dollar salary, living an amazing life with choice over anything and everything I want?

As far as I see it, that mentor sells me money at a discount. I give him $30,000, I get ten times that back. But that isn't how the majority think. They see expense where the millionaires see investment.

Every smart investor knows that you must wait a while for your return after you make the play. In my case, I invested $30,000 with this person and walked out with three or four ideas that I knew I would turn into more than a million dollars in the subsequent next six to twelve months. Sooner, ideally.

It isn't a question of it being expensive, it's just a question of me doing as I am told after having spent the money to get the guy's advice. I'm confident enough in myself to know that I will.

Now you might be thinking, *But there's no way I could afford $30,000 at this stage*. And nor could I when I was at the beginning of my entrepreneurial journey. But I could re-route the money that I was spending on things that really didn't make that much difference to my life at the time. Stuff like clothes, jewelery, meals in expensive restaurants. I questioned why I was buying all of that and made the decision to stop and invest my money instead.

I even made the decision to press pause on buying my dream home.

True story: I'd saved up nearly $100,000 over a few years of being a very in-demand physical therapist, running a very successful physical therapy business in the North East of England.

I had the money to buy it, but I knew that if I bought that house, which we were renting at the time with a view to buying, I wouldn't have much left over for investing in myself or the business.

So, I had a *somewhat* difficult conversation with Natalie that turned out to be one of the best. It went something like this, "Honey, I know you love this dream home, that is perfect for the kids, but can we *not* buy it so that I can spend all the money we saved on business coaching and masterminds, that also happen to be in the USA" (we lived in the UK at the time).

If she had *three* eyebrows, Natalie would have raised them all.

Anyway, she "agreed" that masterminds and coaching was a better use of the money, and we decided *not* to buy the house at the time and rented somewhere smaller instead.

We didn't have the dream house, but it meant I had a bit more money available and instead of buying a new car, fancy clothes, or a watch—or holidaying extravagantly with it—I invested it in business coaching, seminars, and joining peer group-type masterminds to advance my thinking and business skills.

I remember one year quite vividly. I spent all the six figure profits from my physical therapy business on business coaching. When my accountant asked me where all the money had gone, I told him I'd invested it in *myself*. I'll never forget his face. He thought I was stupid.

A few years later when I'd made over a million dollars profit in *one year*, he would go on to ask me for *my* advice on how to market *his* business and charge more for *his* services. I told him I'd happily consult with him—for a fee. But he wasn't keen on paying the price.

GET YOUR ACHIEVEMENT BOOK RESOURCE KIT: WWW.EXABOOK.COM/FREE

There he was, staring at the results of my investment, visibly aware of the success I'd made of my business from taking and getting advice from smart people, but he was still unable to bring himself to pay for the same thing. I know his business has remained stuck at the same level for more than a decade and not much will ever change.

Until *he* does, that is.

"Comfortably Poor"

This, I am sad to say, doesn't surprise me and kind of sums up why so many people get stuck and remain stuck. Especially in businesses. They are mostly unhappy with where they are, but *not* so uncomfortable that they would ever risk time and money of their own to change it. "Comfortably poor" is the phrase. It is everywhere.

Anyway, after that difficult conversation to *not* buy the dream house, a few years later, Natalie is now the owner of multiple dream homes, in multiple countries.

Great things do happen if you make a plan, and you execute on it.

Sometimes you just have to wait a little while for them to arrive. Delayed gratification rather than instant. I do believe that if you can spend a couple of years of your life doing what others won't—investing and growing personally—the prize is spending the rest of your life living how others never could but wish they were: *extraordinarily*.

One more story on this matter: I remember when I first used to leave the UK to fly to the United States to attend these business coaching events I've mentioned in this chapter. I did it so frequently that it felt like I was there every month.

Truth is, many times I was!

I hated leaving the kids. And each time I did, I would ask Natalie *not* to tell my boys (when they inevitably asked where I was), that I was at work.

That would be too easy. Besides, I wasn't. I was off having fun in America learning how to grow a business. But seriously, I wanted to apply a different *meaning* to my absence, one much better than "work."

Instead of "work," I asked her to tell my boys that I've *gone to get another tile for the swimming pool in our next home*. A metaphor for what was happening in my head.

See, every piece of new information, strategy, or idea I got from every seminar I attended was equivalent to a new *tile* for the new swimming pool I was building in my mind that my boys would one day be swimming in. We didn't have the house or the pool, but in my head we already did, I just needed to do the work to make it a reality.

See, a house with a swimming pool was something I'd always dreamed of as a kid, as was living in America, and I knew that one day we would own one if I kept on learning about myself and developing my business skills. To no surprise to me, both came true.

These days, when people come to my house and get in that swimming pool in sunny Orlando, Florida, I can't help but wonder what life would have been like had I not made that investment in myself. I often wonder just how much fun we would be missing out on had I *not* gotten up at 4 AM to fly from England to Chicago and attend that first seminar I paid a few thousand dollars for.

What's funny is that when I was growing up as a kid in the UK, I used to *hate* Sundays. Especially at 6 PM, in the middle of winter, when my mother would shout it was time for getting in the bath and ready for school the next day. It signalled the end of my weekend and all my fun over for another five days.

These days, at 6 PM every Sunday at my house in Florida, I get my boys ready for a swim in the *pool* and let them play as long as they want. That's their equivalent of my bath time. It's also another rule I love "violating."

On a serious note, it's things like this that remind me how far we've come and that the investment has been worth every penny. It's a way of living that is beyond what is possible in the *ordinary* world of survival and compliance. It's a way of living that goes beyond rule following and taking life so seriously and it is only made possible when you do the work *on yourself.*

Anyway, that's enough of my romanticizing about my life in Orlando.

I want you to know that I share these stories not to brag in any way, but because I want to remind you that although tempting to think so, it's not just you who is faced with these types of big decisions about the future. These types of conversations are going on in the homes of most of the entrepreneurs that you admire, every day, every night.

I am sure that at some point, if not right now, you will have to make a similar big decision that involves risk or investing money into your business and I also bet you wish you knew that it wasn't just happening to you.

Well, that's why I share my stories.

It's to make you feel a bit better, to know that what you're going through is normal (in the world of prosperity and opportunity) and is not just happening to you. If you avoid the decisions, you'll probably stay stuck and where you are. Fine if you're happy, but I suspect if you're still reading this far into the book, you probably want more.

And rightly so. Good for you.

I want you to know that you're not alone, what you're going through is common, and you're probably on the right track with whatever you are thinking. Have the courage to see it through, inspired by knowing that others are doing the same things and making similar big decisions.

The rest of the world might not agree with you, but you probably don't want their lives, so why would you care? Why would you give anyone who's life you don't want the chance to have a say on the one you're carving out for yourself?

Besides, just wait until they're swimming in your version of the pool in Florida.

They'll soon change their opinion of you. They only issue you'll have is getting rid of them after they've had too much alcohol from lazing by the pool all day.

Major Principle of Chapter 14: The life you want is only made possible by being OK with risk. Get comfortable with investing time and money into your business development and the sky is the limit.

ACHIEVEMENT
CHAPTER 15

The Unreasonable Club

As we come to a close, I'd like to sum up the major points of the book, the foremost being that *life is about enjoying it and feeling good about yourself as you live it.*

To settle for anything less doesn't make any sense to me.

There's simply no point to life if you're not going to at least make the commitment to enjoy it. Don't start with, "How will I make it through?" Instead, start with, "What's great about life right now and where's my next big opportunity?"

Don't think about merely surviving, obsess over *thriving*.

And by thriving, I don't just mean the amount of money you're making or the things you're acquiring. I mean in how great you *feel about yourself* and life in general.

@THEPAULGOUGH

Remind yourself regularly that life isn't a dress rehearsal. You're not going to get another go at it. And just because others are struggling with it, that doesn't mean it's *meant* to be a struggle. How they've chosen to live their lives and how you *can* live yours are two different things. If in doubt, remember what I said in Chapter 11: *zig when they zag.*

Other people *choosing* to see things as problems doesn't mean you can't choose to see the same things as challenges. Others choosing to see life as risky or tough, or hard and difficult, doesn't mean you can't see it as *fun* and *interesting, unpredictable* and *exciting.*

Other people deciding Lady Luck doesn't shine down on them doesn't mean you can't follow Lady Luck on Instagram, drop her a quick message to ask where she's playing today, and then go park your car close by to get in on the action.

How you decide to live your life, well, it really is all up to you.

And that's the real beauty of life.

The ultimate tool that you've got is the ability to see life exactly as you want it to be. If you want to see that you're here to enjoy it, and feel good about yourself, why not start today?

Because if not now, when?

Seriously, if now is not a good time to start enjoying yourself and life, tell me when is? Is it after the kids go back to school? After Christmas? Next year, when a "new you" is miraculously going to show up? I hear that type of thing all the time from business owners but frankly it said by people who speak ambition but have no intention of doing what is required of ambition. I suspect anyone who says something like that has done so more than once and that is why their life always looks the same.

GET YOUR ACHIEVEMENT BOOK RESOURCE KIT: WWW.EXABOOK.COM/FREE

Another key point I raised at the start is of the book is about *money*, and its unquestionable link to enjoying life.

Make no mistake, money is important in this life. However, don't forget that money isn't the absolute guarantee of an extraordinary life that many people seem to think it is. Especially the ones without much of it, I might add.

Having a bit of money does not *guarantee* an amazing life, but the absence of it sure does make life a lot harder. If in doubt, err on the side of caution and make sure you prioritize getting a bit. There aren't many situations in which having a bit more cash won't come in handy. Just watch what you have to give up getting it.

Making money can be quite the thrill, and it's been my experience that counting it can be fun from time to time too—especially if there's nothing good on the TV or I'm a bit bored on a beach somewhere. There are worse ways to sharpen one's own arithmetic skills than to discover the total sum of all your different bank accounts added together.

However, I also believe that life isn't just about making a lot of money for the sake of getting it or hoarding it, just to say that you're loaded and then think that all your problems will disappear. Nor is it for the purpose of thinking that you're better than others because you've got some.

It may be true that what you had to learn to make the money made you a more *rounded* individual, and gave you a more *rounded* view of life, with a *different* outlook on life to most, but it doesn't make you "better."

This reminds me, there's a guy on my street with a fair bit of money and a top-of-the-range Lamborghini. He might have a bit more money and a better car than most, but he's a real *asshole*. Never smiles either. Even when he's in it. I'd like to have a drive of his car to pick up my coffee one morning, but I wouldn't want him in it with me.

He has the car, possibly the money, but he takes life far too seriously for my liking. He's really boring and his wife is a bit grim also. Loads of money, an expensive watch and plenty of Botox, but not a smile between either of them.

(Perhaps there's too much Botox?)

Just for fun, my fun, I often encourage my boys to kick the soccer ball close to his car, just to set him off! It can be quite entertaining if the ball gets close enough to his drive and it certainly puts an end to his enjoyment of watching Netflix until we go inside.

Anyway, it's also not about making as much money as you can, as some people want you to believe. That's dumb advice because it doesn't factor in what you have to give up while getting it, or if getting it would even make any difference to your life if you did.

It doesn't factor in that as your business gets bigger it will undoubtedly come with more responsibilities and unexpected challenges that will take up more time and simply may not be worth the extra cash relative to what you will lose—such as bedtime stories with kids or being in the gym and keeping healthy.

To have a terrific life—an Extraordinary one—things like this must be considered.

It's really about making as much money as you can, **but *relative* to the quality of life you want the money for in the first place**.

Now that's a smart way to look at it.

@THEPAULGOUGH

I'd like for you to remember that making money is great but it's about so much more than just having it. It's equally about *how you got it* and *how you feel about how you got* it as well as what you had to give up getting it. There's also a lot to be said for what you're going to do with it once you've got it.

As I said earlier in the book, if you're into conscious capitalism, and saving the world with your business, and all that good stuff that looks amazing on your social media bio, you can do lots of good with lots of cash at your disposal. Become a professional philanthropist, perhaps?

And equally, I think it's just as cool to have it to spend as and when *you* want so that you can contribute to the economy buying your own personal yacht, or a Jacuzzi in the bedroom, and keeping people in good jobs because of it.

"They" might say you're being elaborate, or extravagant, even wasteful and unthoughtful. But I'd bet they'd all get in either if you had either. Especially if you had the bubbles turned up in the Jacuzzi and there was a free bottle of wine on the side.

People will try, but do not be guilted into being ashamed of wanting money or enjoying the benefits of it. They're all *at it* in one way or the other. Even the new saviors of the world, Meghan Markle and Prince Harry. They love to spout about saving the world and sorting out climate change etc.—*so long as* you pay them $1,000,000 to show up and cover the cost of the private jet to get there, that is.

Call me cynical, *but*….

Remember it's usually the ones *without money* who will judge you for your pursuit of it. However, they're also the same people lining up to play the weekly Powerball or Mega Millions lottery hoping to get in on the action, so don't take their opinion all that seriously or to heart. It will soon change when they're in the Bentley dealership test driving a new Continental.

As an aside, you'll know who has and hasn't made a bit of money in this life without even looking at their tax returns. Someone who *has* made it themselves knows exactly what you're going through and the gets the journey you're on, and how hard it is, so will do nothing but encourage and support you. They'll never try to put or pull you down as they always want you to join them.

The other thing is when you've made a bit of money, don't go out of your way to make it obvious you're loaded, but equally don't hide it. That's like telling yourself you've done something wrong. You're creating and consuming your own guilt if you do.

If they ask, tell them. If you've got it, drive it or fly in it! Besides, you never quite know who you're going to inspire with that photo of you and your kids flying in a private jet to a big sporting event posted all over social media.

Two types of people look at the same photo: one is envious and wants to press the "asshole" button but settles for the "like" button, albeit through very gritted teeth.

Then there's the second type, the one who looks at the picture of the champagne popping on take-off and thinks, *Good for you. I would love to do that and now if you can do it, so can I. I'm going for it next.* Same photo, same event, two different reactions but ultimately one choice.

Your Invitation To Join The "Unreasonable Club"

@THEPAULGOUGH

In the pages of this book, I've shared with you some of the things that have and continue to work for me. Whether it is a need to break a few rules (Chapter 2), focusing on personal acceptance before personal development (Chapter 3), to stop taking life so seriously (Chapter 5), the importance of energy (Chapter 6), doing more high-leverage work (Chapter 8), making use of leverage (Chapter 9), making big decisions (Chapter 10), not following the crowd (Chapter 11), and even not needing approval from the people around you (Chapter 13), all of these things we've covered have helped me along the way, in some way.

It is a rare book in that it considers both the making of a lot of money and feeling good about yourself at the same time.

I've shared with you my own conviction for each one of these things and, as important as they all are, I think there's one that might just trump the lot. And that is the ability to be completely and absolutely *unreasonable*.

Yes, you read it right, unreasonable.

If there's ever a club that you want to get into, it's the "Unreasonable Club."

And don't feel guilty about joining it either. The world needs more unreasonable people. Remember that all progress is at the hands of unreasonable people.

Now, I'm not suggesting that you be unreasonable all the time—just *most of it*.

Especially when it comes to your happiness, your life, your money, your relationships, your time, your business, and the fun you want to have in life. Be so unreasonable about all those things that people would be forgiven for thinking your life depends upon them.

Truth is, it probably does.

Certainly the type of life I've spoken about in this book where you're autonomous, independent, and free to live, think, and feel as you wish. If you want anything that resembles that type of life, you will not get it being reasonable about important things.

I want to encourage you to be *unreasonable* about demanding more fun in your life. Be *unreasonable* about how much you will accept as payment for services in your business. Be *unreasonable* about who you spend time with and about what you will let them talk about. Be *unreasonable* about standards in your office, the work ethic of the people you're paying, as well as the latest crazy fad of letting staff work from home.

If you like the idea of paying ten people when all you needed was eight to do the same job, then let all your staff work from home. It might be popular since COVID, but it's the death of productivity and the beginning of the inmates running the asylum if you give in to it.

The other thing you must commit to is being *unreasonable* in your demands for *yourself* and of others whose lives stand to benefit from you doing so—even if they don't know it yet and even if they might dislike it at first.

Basically, what I'm saying is to be *unreasonable* in any which way you can.

Leave nothing to chance. And if ever you think you're starting to be a bit *too* reasonable, that you're becoming a bit too tolerant of things and people's drama, I recommend you go on some kind of "unreasonable spree" and behave so unreasonably that people start asking you why you are suddenly being so unreasonable.

When they do, simply tell them it's because it's been too long since anyone called you unreasonable, or accused you of it, and because of that that you're making up for lost time. Tell them that you need to hear that you're being unreasonable at least twice a day before you're happy you've rediscovered your unreasonableness "mojo."

That should be enough to restore an appropriate level of unreasonableness to your life at the same time as giving yourself a good laugh as you watch the looks on the faces of people around you as you explain your goal for the week. Especially your in-laws. And especially that *twit* from the HOA who won't let you paint the front door light pink.

Take it as a given that if you aren't making unreasonable demands of yourself, of others, of your business and its ability to produce the type of money that makes being in business worthwhile, at best, you will get stuck at the average level of life where all of the frustration in life is found.

I didn't write this book to encourage you to be average and I'm sure you didn't pick it up with the hope of living that way either.

Being reasonable might be nice for harmony, for being liked, and for getting along with everyone you meet, and all that stuff reasonable people with reasonable salaries and reasonable opportunities in life like to do. Which is fine, if that's the goal of your life.

But if at any time you want more than an average salary, average house, or an average amount of choices available to you, you will have to be OK with being deemed at least a little bit unreasonable in the eyes of the people around you.

Highlight this next part: *you can't be reasonable and rich.*

You can be accepting and do "OK" but if you want more, you will have to ruffle a few feathers to get what you want. If you want to be rich, in monetary terms *and* quality of life, you will need to be unreasonable and that will mean you'll annoy or disappoint a few people in the process.

But don't worry, when you get there—rich—they'll all forgive you for fear of missing out on a piece of the action. When you're unreasonable and broke, you're an asshole.

However, when you're unreasonable and *rich*, that's a different story. You did what you had to do, and all is forgiven. Watch out, they're a fickle bunch out there.

One final, important point on this: yes, be unreasonable, but don't be so unreasonable that it makes you *un*happy. The key is to be "unreasonable on demand." Do not make it a permanent state you live in. Do it just enough to ensure that you are happy and are getting what you want, making the progress that you need.

Be unreasonable, but not miserable.

Basically, use it, don't let it use you. See it as a tool that you can pick up whenever you need to start making a few changes or speeding up the process of getting what you want.

Did I Offend Anyone?

We're almost at the end of the book and as I wrap up the writing of it, I am conscious that this book doesn't exactly comply with conventional or traditional views of life that are widely accepted by the masses.

Who knows, it may one day even be worthy of "cancelling." (Gasp!)

 GET YOUR ACHIEVEMENT BOOK RESOURCE KIT: WWW.EXABOOK.COM/FREE

Surely, in this day and age, where the *powers that be* are more into control and coercion, poverty and surviving, any book that is about giving people back their own power, openly promotes free and independent thinking, and encourages the use of one's own mind, not to mention the making of *lots* of money, is surely going to offend someone and is therefore at risk of being cancelled?

Well, I do hope so! (I did promise in the introduction that I would at least try!)

I do hope that it offends at least a few people enough to write and let me know (contact details at the end) just how deeply offended they are at my views on life, success, being happy and the making of lots of money.

I am a lonesome entrepreneur and aside from soccer with my kids, I don't get out that much, and so a few irate emails serve as some welcome entertainment as well as a handy reminder not to take life too seriously.

I'm expecting at least one email about the golf course story, and probably one or two about my parenting skills. And if not about either, surely there'll be a complaint about my imaginative portrayal of the modern-day Elders governing the world with fear in the same way as they did in the 1500s?

Or perhaps it'll be from someone whose high heels have just broken and doesn't like me poking fun at the idea of someone trying to fix that same shoe by bashing it in the floor?

Who knows, but I wait with bated breath.

And by the way, if you didn't like the book, if nothing else, at least you will have learned something about the good-old English sense of humor (you did notice some of my jokes, didn't you?) as well as one or two new British phrases you could introduce to your kids after reading this (i.e., "a few Bob," "Cat amongst the pigeons," and "Twit").

Anyway, *Paul*, back to it.

Yes, this book is obviously a "little" anti-political or anti-society (*understatement of the year!*), and the sweeping generalizations I make about "the masses" can be seen as a little derogatory. I know that. I am aware of how some of the things I say *could* be perceived and what I've said *could* irritate a few billion people if this book was in the wrong hands.

Chances are it won't, though.

It would mean spending time and money on something other than food and TV which they're unlikely to do. *Ouch!*

I appreciate I am a little "far out" sometimes. I'm a *lot* weird, I'm definitely candid, have a *no bull-shit* attitude, have very little patience for mediocrity or excuses, and I'm a little opinionated, or maybe a lot opinionated, depending upon *your* opinion. However, I'm also determined to live *my* life, even if it means a few people disliking it or me.

To help, I came to the conclusion early on that what other people do in *their lives* is none of my business. Equally, what other people think of me, what I do, and how I live, is also none of *my* business.

I don't know everything.

In fact, I know very little in relative terms, all things considered. But what I do know is that what I've shared in this book works for *me*. I am not in any way trying to sell you on my views of how to live. Far from it, and I have no reason to do so—not in exchange for a measly thirty dollars.

My only intention is to share the *conviction* I have for how these things have improved my life in the hope that others can enjoy life like I am. What you do next is 100 hundred percent up to you. Some of my thoughts and principles might prove useless to you.

They might even make you irate.

They might violate all your beliefs about what life should be like, or what is right and wrong, based upon what you believe or want to believe is true. That's fine. But remember that all of what I've written comes from *my* pursuit of a life that is one that I can call my own. I have a very different goal for my life than most and therefore how I think, how I act, and how I get there, is going to be *different*.

It's why the only difference between this being a great book and a bad book is the goal you have for your life. If you want a 9-5 job, you love to conform to rules and want to take life seriously because you think worrying and being uptight all the time is the best way to stay alive, you will give this book a one-star review.

However, if you want something different, something that resembles more fun, more autonomy and more cash to boot, you may consider giving it *more than one read* not to mention a five-star review on Amazon as it will have contained at least *some* truths that you needed to hear.

If your goal is to live a life that is fulfilled, autonomous, has more good days than bad, and has you feeling like you're somewhat in control of how you feel about it all—as well as making a good bit of money along the way—then everything that I've shared *could* come in handy at some point as you go about your journey.

In that respect, it is not a curriculum to be consumed once. It is more of a guidebook to be referred to from time to time. Keep this in the top draw of the bedside table and take it on vacation with you from time to time. I will bet many of the things I've said will mean more to you as life plays out over the years and you'll have a deeper understanding of each one of these things we've covered as the years go by.

One thing I guarantee is that you will be able to see all the major things—the principles—I've written about in the chapters much more obviously than you ever did. Especially the one about people taking *life too seriously.*

Open Facebook or just look out the window for proof of that. Pay particular attention to the guy wearing a suit so tight he can barely breathe, and especially that lady smashing her recently broken high heel into the floor hoping to fix it. *Lol!*

Balance Ambition and Self-Acceptance

As I said at the start of this 90,000+ word book, in my eyes, Extraordinary Achievement—the title of this book—is **getting what you want, enjoying your life, and feeling good about yourself as you live it**.

It's about making a bit of money along the way that allows you to experience the finer things in life and it's about being prepared to stand up for what you believe in and how you want to live despite and not in spite of others who disagree. Even if you run the risk of being labelled "unreasonable."

I might add that it's about sharing your story and your journey with the ones who ask how you did it. If people are capable of being inspired or want to make progress, they'll show up and ask you how you did it. Most won't, but one or two will.

Resist the temptation to believe it's your obligation to impress upon them how they should live. It's not. They might ask, and if they do want to know how you did it, or how you got what you got, make sure you give it to them after first *billing them* appropriately to learn.

Really, the trick to money is getting some of it and the best way to get it is to *ask*.

(Teach them how to do the same, too.)

Other than that, it's about getting on and doing your thing, not giving two hoots about who is watching or what they're thinking. Don't be intentionally reckless—as if hurting others is the only way to get what you want—and don't piss people off just to feel good or powerful because you can. And definitely don't end up like the guy in my street with the Lambo' who forgot how to smile the day after selling his business (or getting married—I can't decide which one.)

That said, you must be prepared for a little bit of collateral damage and a lot of conflict along the way. How you deal with this conflict, as I said in the earlier part of the book, really could define the quality of your life.

Remember that life is *not* about conforming to stupid, outdated rules. It's *not* about living so seriously that you never laugh unless you're drunk or at the Laugh Out Loud studios in Los Angeles, and it's definitely *not* about working eighteen hours per day thinking you'll get rich if you do so for twenty years.

It's *not* about following the crowd, it's *not* about avoiding big decisions in case people think badly of you or you get it wrong, and it's *not* about finding work/life balance or seeking approval from your parents. It's *not* about pleasing people, being a perfectionist, or even reasonable and loved by everyone for being that way.

It's *none* of that.

The point of life is to enjoy it and feel good about yourself for doing so.

And ideally, make a "few bob" along the way so you can enjoy the finer things in life that are to be savored (that's a British phrase for getting loaded and making more money than you'll ever need.)

I know it's so easy to get consumed by the news of the day, the latest fad, a social movement that promises to change the world for the better—*this time*—and all that type of stuff that it's easy to forget that you're here to live your own life.

The best thing you can do is just that—live your own life. That is ultimately what every person alive wants today. They want the safety and security that comes with the ability to think and act for *themselves*.

I am certain you do too, or you wouldn't *still* be reading this book.

Sure, there are a lot of people out there who really *do* need the help of good causes, noble people, and even the government. But that isn't what this book is about. It's not about saving the world or creating a "movement" or anything else of that nature. I'll leave that to Harry and Meghan.

I am brazen in saying that this book is about **you** (and me!), and **you** (and me!) making the most of the opportunity of a lifetime—that being the opportunity to live a fantastic life you can call your own.

Once you get that, do with it what you wish. All things being equal, the only real challenge you face, especially as an entrepreneur, is balancing your ambition with personal acceptance. That is the one and only game you're playing from here on in.

It's not a question of "Can you make money?" or "Can you be happier from time to time?" It's about balancing them both in pursuit of more of both. Which, if you're an entrepreneur, you're probably going to spend your whole life doing from now until the day you die.

There will always be someone who has made more money, but are they really happy? And there's always going to be someone who is perhaps on the surface happier, but has limited life experiences and frustrated somewhat because they couldn't afford to go out or do anything.

Hunkering down at home every night might be nice, and sure, you can be content doing that, but there must be at least a hint of frustration at never getting to see the world and all it has to offer.

Watching other people on a sunset safari or swimming with sharks in South Africa on TV is nowhere near as fun or exhilarating as doing it yourself. I've done both. The problem is they both require a lot more money than the price of a cable TV subscription.

What I'm saying is the journey isn't one or the other—happy *or* rich—it's how you get the right amount of *both* to be able to say the journey was worth the effort.

Far from work/life balance, it's the one about managing your entrepreneurial ambition and at the same time being OK with *who you are right now* that is going to define the quality of your life, and how you feel as you live your life. It's OK to want more, but not if it's at the price of wasting today thinking everything in the future will be better when you get it.

However you feel right now, it could be better, it could be worse. It could be amazing, it could be awful. It could be secure, it could be insecure. The best news is that you get to decide which one is for you.

Really, that's the only control that you've ever wanted in life—to decide how you feel about yourself—and the good news is that the ability to do so is free, available to you right now, and that same *control* can last as long as you want.

Final, *Final* Thoughts

Anyway, we're *almost* done. But don't dare go anywhere just yet. Before I finish, I want to leave you with these final thoughts that *might*, just *might*, sum up this entire book for you in a few paragraphs. I'm sorry I had to put you through 90,000+ words to get to this point, but I do hope I've provided at least bit of light-hearted entertainment on the way to getting here that made it worthwhile. Anyway, here it is—the final point:

People are hardwired to think and feel a certain way and no politician, social movement, or advancement in technology will ever change that, no matter how much they wish it were true. Technology changes, tools and equipment are advancing and constantly change, and even the social landscape changes according to the narrative of the those who shout the *loudest*. But human nature never changes.

If you're looking for any truth in life, this is it: **how people think, how they act, and what they want from life does not change and most of us are** united in what we want from it, which is to **enjoy it and feel good about living it.** And if you ask me, anyone who takes the time to figure that out really is rich. By any definition.

To clarify, the above doesn't mean you don't care about those other things or other people, only that you shouldn't care more about them than your own life.

To do so is to give your own life away, and given you only get one life, this probably isn't the best use of it.

Besides, and as I've said many times in this book, you're in a much better position to help others when you've *sorted yourself out first*. If you really do want to help others feel better (about themselves), you owe it to them to fix your own insecurities first.

So there can be no doubt, I firmly believe that what people really want is to feel good about themselves and enjoy making progress in life. I believe people do not want to be "ruled over" or told what to do, or even given freebies and handouts. They just don't know how to live any other way, so *endemic* such a way of living has become.

What people really want is to live an autonomous life, one they can call their own, free to act, think, and *feel* exactly how they want. It's not about being a multi-millionaire—although that is nice—and it's not about waking up every day and expecting that it will always be amazing—that's probably not possible.

However, it *is* possible to have more money than you need to survive, more than you have now, and it is possible to have *more* amazing days than you probably are now, too.

I've presented to you just some of the things I believe in that have helped me live that type of life, one where there's more money and more amazing days than most, where I'm free to think, act, and feel precisely how I want.

If you want anything that resembles that, I sincerely hope these things will do the same for you.

Good luck ☺.

Major Principle of Chapter 15: If you want your life to be about progress and you want to feel progress, you're going to have be OK with being unreasonable. All progress is created by unreasonable people.

FREE BONUS: TWO ADDITIONAL *AUDIO* CHAPTERS

I wanted to write a bit more, but with printing and shipping costs being so high these days (I blame the government!), I had to rein it in a little. I decided it best to record the chapters and put them on a private audio file that you can access at:

WWW.EXABOOK.COM/FREE

- ✓ **Bonus Audio (Chapter 16):** The 7 Habits of Hugely Successful Entrepreneurs

@THEPAULGOUGH

✓ **Bonus Audio (Chapter 17):** What to Focus on Next: 6 Things That Should Get Your Time And Attention After This Book

I've also included some additional resources for you on that page that I believe relevant to the theme of this book—success and achievement. **These include:**

✓ The **Self-Assessment Scorecard**—rate yourself on the principles discussed in this book and find out the areas in which you need to make improvements on to get to that next level of success faster.

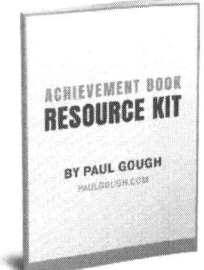

✓ **The Checklist/Poster**—get a copy of all of the principles discussed in one place so you can print it out, put it on your wall and make each one easier to remember and implement into your life.
✓ **Instant Access Video:** Watch me talk about some of these principles LIVE on stage.
✓ **Free Chapters:** Get the first two chapters of my best-selling book *Leadership In Private Practice.*
✓ **Surprise Items:** Plus, at least two other surprise items that if you have enjoyed this book, I know you will love.

Moreover, if you are a **physical therapist** or owner of a **private practice**, I invite you to head over to my website, **www.paulgough.com**, where you can find lots of valuable, but free to use, resources on how to build your private practice and make a lot more money.

On my website (and on iTunes), you will also find my top-rated podcast—**The Paul Gough Podcast and Audio Experience**—that to date has more than one million verified plays.

Yes, that said *one million.*

There is also a **Free 90-Day Marketing Plan** you can get from me and the offer of a free consultation with a member of my marketing team. It will be very valuable to you—especially if you are absent of one at present or the one you have does not work.

Anyhow, well done for reading this far. I sincerely appreciate your interest in my work. I hope we can meet in person one day and discuss how this book has impacted you over a cold beer, coffee, or glass of wine.

Good luck on your journey to finding a life that is *Extraordinary*. Remember that success is about getting what you want, moreover, living an extraordinary life is *considering what you got, how you feel about how you got it and how long it lasts.*

That is next level.

That is what transcends success. That is what this book was all about. I hope you enjoyed reading it as much as I enjoyed writing it.

Best wishes,
Paul Gough

GET YOUR ACHIEVEMENT BOOK RESOURCE KIT: **WWW.EXABOOK.COM/FREE**

@THEPAULGOUGH

Contact me:

paul@paulgough.com

www.paulgough.com

Telephone: +1 407-567-0086

Instagram: @ThePaulGough

YouTube: ThePaulGough

Podcast: The Paul Gough Podcast and Audio Experience (available on iTunes, SoundCloud, Spotify, etc.)

Other best-selling books in the series are available on Amazon and at www.paulgoughbooks.com. Topics include *marketing, hiring, sales, and leadership.*

Private Practice Marketer Live: The biggest marketing and business growth super conference in the world for private practice owners. Past speakers include Daymond John (ABC's *Shark Tank*), Marcus Lemonis (CNBC's *The Profit*), Kevin O'Leary (ABC's *Shark Tank*), Dan Kennedy (Author and worlds best marketer), John Barnes (Liverpool FC), Mike Michalowiz (Author of *Profit First*), and more.

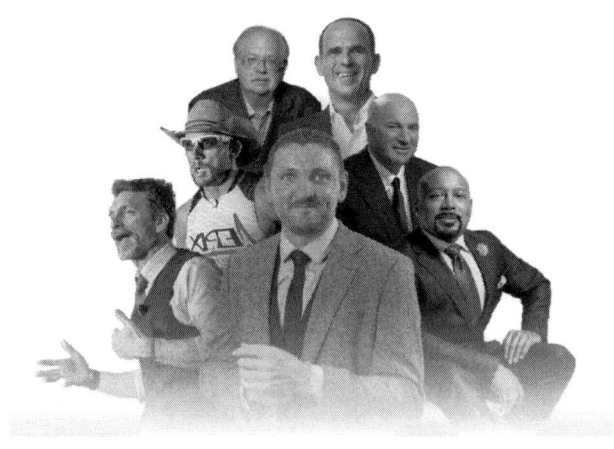

GET YOUR ACHIEVEMENT BOOK RESOURCE KIT: WWW.EXABOOK.COM/FREE

Now You've Finished Reading The Book...

The 2-Day
EXTRAORDINARY ACHIEVEMENT
IN-PERSON WORKSHOP

"If you like what you read in this book, and you want to continue the journey, why not attend the **TOTAL IMMERSION** two-day event and work personally with Paul Gough to implement these life enhancing principles into your life?"

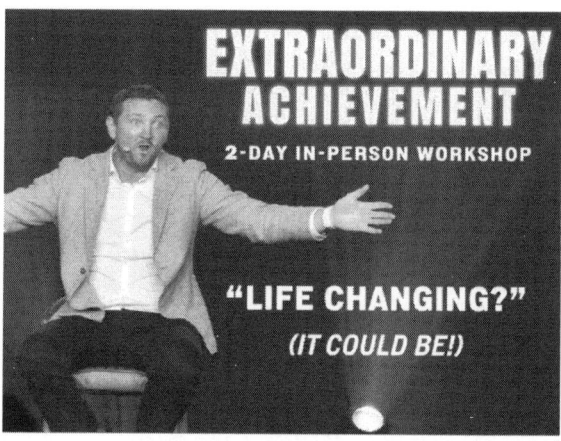

To Find Out When & Where In The World,
Register Your Interest At:

EXABook.com/Workshop
(Email: paul@paulgough.com)

Also By Paul Gough:

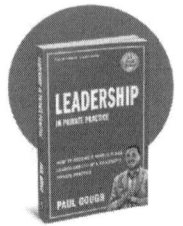

Leadership In Private Practice
"How To Become A World Class Leader And CEO Of A Successful Private Practice"

www.PaulsLeadershipBook.com

New Patient Accelerator Method
"How I Scaled a Four Location, $1,000,000+ Cash-Pay Physical Therapy Clinic – In A Place Where Healthcare Is Free" (… And, in One of the Poorest Areas of the Country)

www.PaulsMarketingBook.com

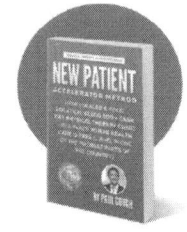

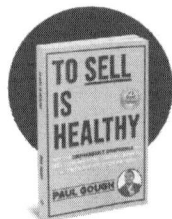

To Sell Is Healthy
"Get The Unshakeable Confidence To Sell Your Physical Therapy Services – At Twice The Price You Are Now"

www.PhysicalTherapySalesBook.com

The Physical Therapy Hiring Solution
"How To Recruit, Hire, And Train World-Class People You Can Trust"

www.PaulsMarketingBook.com

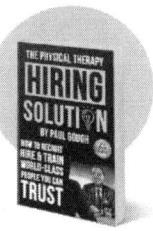

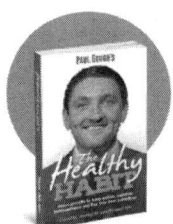

The Healthy Habit
"Learn Secrets To Keep Active, Maintain Independence And Live Free From Painkillers. Essential Reading For People Aged 50+"

www.PaulsLeadershipBook.com

PaulGoughBooks.com

Made in the USA
Columbia, SC
19 April 2025